Younger People with Dementia: A Multidisciplinary Approach

Younger People with Dementia: A Multidisciplinary Approach

Robert Baldwin
and
Michelle Murray
Editors

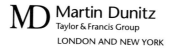
Martin Dunitz
Taylor & Francis Group
LONDON AND NEW YORK

© 2003 Martin Dunitz, an imprint of the Taylor & Francis Group plc

First published in the United Kingdom in 2003 by Martin Dunitz, an imprint of the Taylor and Francis Group plc, 11 New Fetter Lane, London EC4P 4EE

Tel.:   +44 (0) 20 7583 9855
Fax.:   +44 (0) 20 7842 2298
E-mail: info@dunitz.co.uk
Website: http://www.dunitz.co.uk

A CIP record for this book is available from the British Library.

ISBN 1 84184 272 9

Distributed in the USA by
Fulfilment Center
Taylor & Francis
10650 Tobben Drive
Independence, KY 41051, USA
Toll Free Tel.: +1 800 634 7064
E-mail: taylorandfrancis@thomsonlearning.com

Distributed in Canada by
Taylor & Francis
74 Rolark Drive
Scarborough, Ontario M1R 4G2, Canada
Toll Free Tel.: +1 877 226 2237
E-mail: tal_fran@istar.ca

Distributed in the rest of the world by
Thomson Publishing Services
Cheritor House
North Way
Andover, Hampshire SP10 5BE, UK
Tel: +44 (0) 1264 332424
E-mail: salesorder.tandf@thomsonpublishingservices.co.uk

Composition by Wearset Ltd, Boldon, Tyne & Wear
Printed and bound in Great Britain by Biddles Ltd, Guildford and King's Lynn

Contents

Contents

Contributors

Robert Baldwin DM, FRCP, FRCPsych
Consultant Psychiatrist and Honorary Professor of Old Age Psychiatry
Manchester Mental Health and Social Care Trust
York House
Manchester Royal Infirmary
Manchester

Caroline Browne D. CLIN PSY
Trainee Clinical Psychologist
Institute for Health Research
Lancaster University
Lancaster

Catherine Byrne
Support Worker
Younger Persons Dementia Service
Carisbrooke Resource Centre
Manchester

Ruth Chaplin DIP OT, BSc
Senior Occupational Therapist
Younger Persons Dementia Service
Carisbrooke Resource Centre
Manchester

Denise Dickson
Support Worker
Younger Persons Dementia Service
Carisbrooke Resource Centre
Manchester

Kenneth Garrod BA (Econ.), CQSW, Diploma in Counselling
Social Worker, University Teacher
Carisbrooke Resource Centre
Manchester

Jackie Kindell BSc (Hons) Speech
Pathology
Specialist Speech and Language
Therapist
Therapy Office, The Meadows
Stockport

Catherine Kinsella
Support Worker
Younger Persons Dementia Service
Carisbrooke Resource Centre
Manchester

Alice Knight
Trainee Clinical Psychologist
Academic Division of Clinical
Psychology
School of Psychiatry and
Behavioural Sciences
Research Centre,
Wythenshawe Hospital
Manchester

Sally Mendham BA (Hons) App Soc
Studies, CQSW, Alzheimer's Society Approved
Trainer
Project Manager
Stockport Dementia Care Training
Project
Stockport

Michelle Murray RMN, Diploma in
Dementia Care
Specialist Nurse
Younger Persons Dementia Service
Carisbrooke Resource Centre
Manchester

David Neary
Consultant Neurologist and
Professor of Neurology
Cerebral Function Unit
Greater Manchester
Neuroscience Centre
Hope Hospital
Salford
Manchester

Sean Page MSc, BSc (Hons), RMN
DIPN (Lond)
Clinical Nurse Specialist
Memory Clinic
Wythenshawe Hospital
Manchester

Emma Shlosberg D. Clin Psy
Consultant Clinical Psychologist
Department of Clinical
Psychology
Manchester Mental Health and
Social Care Partnership
Manchester Royal Infirmary
Manchester

Julie Snowden
Neuropsychologist
Cerebral Function Unit
Greater Manchester
Neuroscience Centre
Hope Hospital
Salford
Manchester

Preface

Younger people with dementia present a unique challenge to society and to those individuals who care for them. In the minds of many, dementia is a disease of older people with inevitable but unfortunate connotations of senility and decay. It challenges these perceptions when the disease tragically affects younger people.

There is no doubt that services for younger people with dementia have lagged behind those for the elderly, and specialist interest services and professionals, such as those reflected in this book, are few and far between. Numerically, the numbers of younger people with dementia are dwarfed by their older counterparts, but the upset for families, the presence of dependent young children, and the economic implications are amongst the particular challenges. The special part that genetics has to play in the wider management and counselling of younger people with dementia is also important, and many of the advances in molecular biology and the genetics of dementia have been uncovered by investigations of younger families.

Spearheaded by Robert Baldwin and Michelle Murray, this publication aims to provide knowledge and disseminate experience based on practice in caring for younger people with dementia. The authors have pioneered the service in Manchester through traditional commitment and hard work, and this is a service to whose quality I can personally attest. Contributions cover the span of aetiology, multi-professional involvement, support for patient and carers and, uniquely and importantly, the views of service users and their direct carers. Thoughtful and readable chapters convey the enthusiasm and experience of the contributors and have been corralled expertly by the editors into a very readable volume.

This unique and original contribution sets the standard for knowledge and experience in this area.

Alistair Burns, President
International Psychogeriatric Association

Acknowledgements

We would like to acknowledge the advice and support of the following individuals in gathering important information relevant to services for younger people with dementia in Manchester: Jeanette Tilley and Catherine Slough of the Alzheimer's Society; Ian Nixon of HIV City-Wide Liaison Service; Neil Smith, Occupational Therapist working with Manchester Mental Health & Social Trust, and colleagues from the North West Regional Development Forum chaired by Professor Ken Wilson. Last, but by no means least, we thank our service users and their carers for tireless support on behalf of the service.

chapter 1

Introduction

Robert Baldwin and Michelle Murray

This book is about providing a specialist service to younger people who have dementia. Some reports and texts already exist (Cox & Keady, 1999; Royal College of Psychiatrists, 2001; Alzheimer's Society, 2001). What then is new about this book? First, we have given enough factual information that it can be used as a free-standing text on the topic. Second, this is a practical book with a focus on teamwork. We discuss the roles of different professions, describe how the specialist multidisciplinary team functions and suggest ways of networking with other agencies. Those new to the topic will find clinical information about the dementias that occur in younger people and specialists' suggestions about how a team might be developed. Third, we have tried to translate our local experience of service development into suggestions for those planning and commissioning services.

All the contributors work, have worked, or have close links with the Manchester service for younger people with dementia, sometimes known as the 'Carisbrooke service'. Some might see utilizing local experience in these ways as a disadvantage as no two geographical areas are precisely the same. However, we are part of a forum for services in the North West region of England, have strong links with the Alzheimer's Society and, wider still, are abreast with international developments through organizations such as the International Psychogeriatric Association (IPA). We have tried to place our work in this wider context to avoid becoming parochial.

However, in planning this text it became clear that the UK is a leader in this field. We could find no examples of a similar approach to specialist care in other countries. In the United States, unlike the UK, there has been no strategic initiative to develop services for younger people with dementia. Services are provided more on a piecemeal basis usually through two organizations, the American Alzheimer's Association and/or the federally funded National Institute on Aging (NIA) Alzheimer's Disease Centers (ADCs). The American Alzheimer's Association is about to complete a three-year strategic initiative to consolidate some of their smaller chapters, but will emerge with around 100 chapters nationwide of which approximately 20% offer specific support groups for people with early onset dementia and their families. The 29 ADCs located at major medical institutions across the country are the major research centres (besides the Reagan Research Institute of the National Alzheimer's Association) conducting basic clinical, and behavioural research, in addition to training health care providers and helping families to cope. A few of the centres have developed services for disease-specific dementias that most often occur in younger people, such as frontal lobe dementia, but none are specifically designed only for the younger age group (PB Harris, pers. comm., see the References). Thus, we hope that this book will stimulate not only local but also international developments.

How did the Manchester service begin? Following a local survey in 1994 it was found that there were about 150 people within the City of Manchester with a dementia arising between the ages of 18 and 64 years (Baldwin, 1994). The specialist service in Manchester began in 1996 with the identification of one of us (RCB) as the lead psychiatric consultant and the other (MM) as development worker, later to become a specialist nurse. Since then we have expanded so that in addition we have 3.5 whole-time equivalent (wte) community support workers, 0.6 wte senior occupational therapist, 0.2 wte speech and language therapist, 0.1 wte clinical psychologist, 0.1 wte physiotherapist and 0.5 wte social worker. Our physical resource, Carisbrooke Research Centre, permits a maximum of 10 attendees per day for day care four days a week plus one evening session every other week and daily outreach into the home. In addition, we offer specialist assessments of younger people with dementia but we do not offer a diagnostic service. This is conducted prior to referral by the referrer or through the local Memory Clinic or the specialist Cerebral Function Unit based in the Neurology Department. The latter two cover the City of Manchester and beyond and are based in neighbouring hospitals. Both are described in this book (Chapters 2 and 12).

Although dementia occurs much less commonly in younger than older people, it is estimated that there are about 17,000 affected younger people in the UK (Alzheimer's Society, 2001). For those between the ages of 30 and 64 years, this translates to 67 cases per 100,000 with Alzheimer's disease alone in a given locality. These numbers are sufficient to justify specific recognition in planning and service provision, especially given the results of a number of surveys which show that those affected do not readily fit into existing health and social care systems.

Importantly, the range of disorders differs in younger people. Figure 1.1 shows the proportions of the main forms of dementias that affect this age group (Alzheimer's Society, 2001). So although Alzheimer's disease and vascular dementia (VaD) remain the most common types

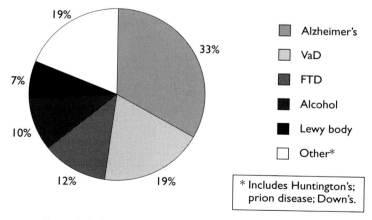

Figure 1.1 *Prevalence of dementias in younger adulthood.*

of dementia across all age groups, disorders such as frontotemporal dementia (FTD), Huntington's disease, prion disorders, HIV dementia and dementia in Down's syndrome occur regularly in this age group but are very rare among older adults.

We begin with an overview of the dementias that affect younger adults from two of the leading experts in the field with whom our service has had close links since its inception. Next, we consider assessment, using the skills of our 'core' team members: specialist nurse, psychiatrist, occupational therapist and speech and language therapist. Management incorporates an overview of pharmacological treatment, focusing on cholinesterase inhibitors, which have become emblematic of a more positive view of management of AD, and about which patients and their caregivers require up-to-date information. However, a comprehensive understanding of the roles of psychologist, occupational therapist, speech and language therapist, social worker and community support workers will result, we believe, in the delivery of optimal treatment. These are discussed in detail, but we go further. We are fortunate in having links with a local Old Age Psychiatry family therapy service which we describe in relation to our work with families. We believe that supportive care for both the caregiver and the identified patient is vital. Members of the team present their experience in running support groups in our service. Listening to the views of younger people and their caregivers is not a luxury but a necessity if services are to be responsive to need, and we present data provided by our service users. Finally, no specialist service can stand in isolation. Indeed, the Carisbrooke service is underpinned by our view that younger people with dementia should have exactly the same rights of access to mainstream services as anyone else. Hence, we describe how links can be formed with the local Memory Clinic, an ever more important resource, which facilitates entry to services without stigma, such as social care agencies, HIV and alcohol services, volunteer groups and the local Old Age Psychiatry services. As well as being a source of referral it is important to have agreed protocols with the latter so that smooth transfer can take place if an age-related policy is operated. Throughout, we have used case histories (made anonymous) to illustrate points.

Lest we have not convinced the reader of the need for specialist services, we list below 10 points summarized by the Alzheimer's Society (2001).

Everyone, irrespective of their age, should be entitled to quality support and services that meet all their needs. Younger people with dementia are a significant minority with specific needs and circumstances. This makes a strong case for their specific recognition and provision in service planning.

1 Dementia under the age of 65 is rare and is less likely to be specifically recognized or addressed by services. This causes a considerable additional burden for younger people with dementia and their carers as they are unclear about where to access the support they need.
2 Dementia has an impact on the whole family. However, in families where someone develops dementia under the age of 65, there are specific needs to be addressed. Younger people are more likely to have children and financial commitments dependent on the earnings of the person with dementia and their carer. A person may be forced to leave work to care for his/her partner.
3 There is a higher prevalence of the rarer dementias in younger people. Services need the awareness and experience to work with the different needs presented by the whole range of dementias.
4 The emotional impact of developing dementia at a young age needs to be addressed. For both the person with dementia and their families the diagnosis has a dramatic effect on future life plans and expectations.
5 It has proved difficult to provide a service that meets the individual needs of each person with dementia where the group has a diverse range of needs. For example, younger people are likely to be physically stronger, have work-related aspirations and be of a different generation to the majority of people with dementia.
6 Services should provide an opportunity for mutual support in an environment where people feel at ease. Where services are

designed for older people, they often lack such opportunities for younger people who can feel isolated.

7 Younger people with dementia, their families and friends need different forms of information and emotional support.

8 The impact on staff providing support to younger people with dementia is frequently underestimated. The different and unfamiliar range of needs, the emotional impact of caring for someone of a similar age and the training implications warrant specific consideration.

9 The issues facing younger people with dementia and their families are complex and may change rapidly. There is a need for ongoing specialist involvement and monitoring.

10 Studies have shown a significant risk of carer burden where the needs of younger people with dementia have been overlooked and little or no consideration given to service provision or support.

References

Alzheimer's Society (2001) *Younger People with Dementia: a Guide to Service Development and Provision*. London: Alzheimer's Society (UK).

Baldwin RC (1994) Acquired cognitive impairment in the presenium. *Psychiatr Bull* **18:** 463–465.

Cox S, Keady J (1999) *Younger People with Dementia: Planning, practice and development*. London/Philadelphia: Jessica Kingsley.

Harris PB. Professor of Sociology, Director of Aging Studies Program, John Carroll University, 20700 North Park Blvd., Cleveland, OH 44118, USA. Phone: 216-397-4634; Fax: 216-397-4376.

Royal College of Psychiatrists (2001) *Services for Younger People with Alzheimer's Disease and Other Dementia*. Council Report CR77. London: Royal College of Psychiatrists.

chapter 2

Causes of dementia in younger people

David Neary and Julie Snowden

Dementia is not the name of a disease. It is a descriptive term that describes the mental changes that accompany a variety of different diseases. The most common forms of dementia are degenerative, resulting from intrinsic changes to brain neurons. However, dementia may also occur secondary to vascular disease or may have extrinsic causes. Differentiation between the diverse conditions that give rise to dementia is increasingly important for a number of reasons. First, different diseases are likely to require different remedies. With the advent of new dementia therapies accurate diagnosis is imperative. Second, dementia sometimes runs in families and some diseases are more likely to be familial than others. An accurate diagnosis is vital for appropriate counselling of family members who may be at risk from developing the disease. Third, dementia syndromes are not identical. Different diseases give rise to different patterns of symptoms, reflecting the distribution of the pathological changes within the brain. Understanding the precise manner in which cognition and behaviour are altered by disease helps recognition of individual needs and allows prediction of the future course of disease. It therefore provides the basis for optimal management of dementia sufferers.

Classification of dementia syndromes

Dementia has traditionally been defined as a 'global impairment of intellect', the implication being that all aspects of cognitive function are equally affected and deteriorate in an undifferentiated way. This is not so. Cerebral diseases do not affect the brain uniformly, but preferentially affect certain brain regions and spare others. Moreover, cognitive functions are regionally organized and depend on the functioning of specific brain regions. It follows logically that different cerebral diseases will be associated with distinct and characteristic neuropsychological syndromes, reflecting the specific parts of the brain that are particularly affected by the disease process. An assumption that still prevails is that accurate diagnosis can only be achieved by pathological examination of brain tissue postmortem. While it is certainly true that a definitive diagnosis depends on pathological verification it is also the case that identification of the pattern of cognitive change, together with the pattern of neurological symptoms and signs, can lead to a high level of diagnostic accuracy in life.

A useful method of classifying brain disorders that lead to dementia is on the basis of the parts of the brain predominantly affected by disease (Table 2.1). Some disorders chiefly affect the cortex whereas others predominantly affect subcortical structures. Other diseases involve both cortical and subcortical structures. Only a minority has a multifocal distribution without respect for functional anatomical systems.

The cerebral cortex is critically important for cognition (broadly, our faculties and how we regulate them) (Figure 2.1). These are now briefly discussed. The ability to make sense of what is perceived through the senses is highly dependent on the posterior parts of the cortex. This includes the ability to recognize objects and faces, to appreciate the spatial relationship between external objects and the individual and to understand language. Object recognition (impairment of which causes 'agnosia') is particularly dependent on ventral pathways between occipital and temporal lobes and spatial abilities on parietal regions. Language (impairment of which causes 'aphasia')

Table 2.1 Causes of dementia and their classification

Cortical
- Alzheimer's disease
- Frontotemporal lobe degeneration
  - frontotemporal dementia
  - progressive aphasia
  - semantic dementia
  - progressive apraxia
- Alcoholic dementia

Subcortical
- Progressive supranuclear palsy
- Parkinson's disease
- Huntington's disease
- Vascular dementia
  - subcortical arteriosclerosis
  - CADASIL
- Multiple sclerosis
- Leukodystrophies

Corticosubcortical
- Dementia with Lewy bodies
- Corticobasal degeneration
- Vascular dementia

Multifocal
- Creutzfeldt–Jakob disease

CADASIL, cerebral autosomal dominant arteriopathy with subcortical infarcts and leukoencephalopathy

is dependent on the areas around the sylvian fissure, extending from the frontal into the parietal and temporal lobes in the left hemisphere, the temporal lobe being particularly important for word meaning ('semantics'). Parietal regions of the left hemisphere have an important role in calculation skills. The premotor and superior parietal areas are important for the organization of skilled movements (praxis). The

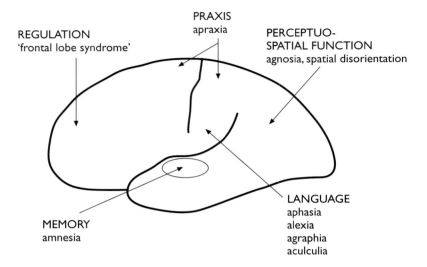

Figure 2.1 *Functional topography of the cerebral cortex. The figure shows psychological syndromes arising from damage to particular brain regions.*

medial portion of both hemispheres, designated the limbic system, which includes the hippocampus and amygdala, is essential for the acquisition and retention of information. Alzheimer's disease is the prototypical disease that affects the posterior and medial parts of the cortex (Figure 2.2).

The posterior and medial parts of the brain are particularly important for the 'tools' of cognition: language, object perception, spatial skills and memory. These aspects of cognition are sometimes referred to as 'instrumental' abilities. The anterior parts of the brain, by contrast, are essential for 'executive' skills, the ability to regulate mental life, which includes strategic planning and purposive, goal-directed behaviour, organization, sequencing and monitoring of actions taking place over time. Breakdown in regulatory processes leads to aberrant personal and social behaviour, change in personality and an inability to conceive of and successfully achieve behavioural goals (dysexecutive syndrome). Frontotemporal dementia is the prototypical disorder that affects the anterior cerebral cortex (Figure 2.2).

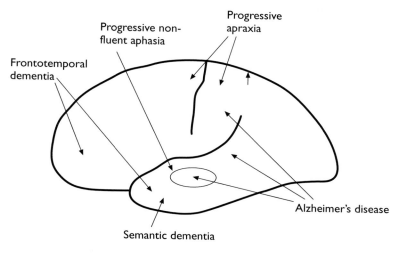

Figure 2.2 *Topographical distribution of impaired function in cortical degenerative disorders.*

Subcortical regions have a critical role in neurological function. Whereas people with cortical diseases have marked cognitive change with relatively few physical problems, in people with subcortical disease the reverse is the case. Thus, in subcortical forms of dementia the mental changes accompany striking physical abnormalities. In disorders that affect both cortex and subcortex the cognitive changes of cortical dementias are combined with the cognitive and physical changes of subcortical disease.

Cortical dementias

Alzheimer's disease

Alzheimer's disease (AD) is the most common degenerative disorder leading to dementia. It is often thought of as a disease of the elderly, and it is certainly true that the prevalence of AD increases with advancing age. Nevertheless, AD can also occur in younger people, beginning in the fourth, fifth or sixth decade of life. Indeed, it is the most common form of dementia in younger people. It is more prevalent in woman than men. The duration of illness is variable ranging from 2 to 16 years, with an average of about 8 years.

Clinical characteristics

The earliest symptom is usually memory failure, particularly for day-to-day events. People may forget appointments, forget to make intended purchases in the supermarket, or forget where they have parked the car. They may be repetitive in conversation. They may show difficulty in learning new information, such as how to use a new household appliance. In the initial stages, forgetfulness may be difficult to distinguish from the memory lapses to which everyone is prone. It is the frequency and persistence of memory failures that alert families to a more sinister underlying problem. With progression of disease there is gradual worsening of memory leading to total disorientation in time and place and severe memory impairment for earlier events.

Memory loss can involve a person's entire lifespan. Nevertheless, information from the distant past may be better preserved than for the recent past. It is for this reason that people in the moderate stages of AD may have a tendency to talk about their youth rather than the present or seem to believe themselves to be at an earlier stage of their life. People who wander may assert that they are 'going home', based on the belief that they are still living in the home of their youth. Memory problems in AD reflect pathological changes in medial temporal lobe structures. In some people, memory loss remains a relatively selective problem for many years before other cognitive deficits emerge, reflecting a circumscribed distribution of pathological change within these brain regions. However, in most people there is spread of pathology to neocortical areas and this is associated with the presence of additional cognitive deficits.

A characteristic feature of Alzheimer's disease is visuospatial impairment, which arises because of involvement of parietal cortex. Spatial problems lead people to become lost in their surroundings, because they no longer have an internal 'spatial map' of the relationship between one place (e.g. the local shops) and another (e.g. the person's home). They may have difficulty orienting clothing when dressing and aligning cutlery when laying a table. They may have difficulty going up and down stairs, because of poor judgement of the spatial depth of each stair and they may trip on kerbstones. Severe spatial problems mean that people may become disoriented even within their own home, so that they no longer know where, for example, the bathroom is in relation to the bedroom. They may be slow to localize objects, so may appear not to 'see' objects placed in front of them. Perceptual impairments generally emerge relatively late in the disease course, and lead to failure of face recognition, including the mirror reflection of the person's own face, and misidentification of objects. Spatial problems typically outweigh perceptual problems in the early and middle phase: patients have difficulty locating objects in the environment, but when once located are recognized accurately.

Language skills are compromised when areas around the perisylvian fissure (Figure 2.1) are affected. Utterances are halting, reflecting word-finding difficulty and people have difficulty maintaining a line of thought so sentences are often unfinished. Comprehension is affected, particularly for complex syntactic sentences. Problems in spelling and calculation are common and are often early features. As the disease progresses, speech output may have a stuttering quality, reflecting spread of pathology into subcortical structures. Breakdown of skilled movements of the arms and legs may occur secondary to spatial disorientation, which results in difficulty copying drawings (constructional apraxia) and dressing (dressing apraxia). Sometimes, however, motor executive difficulties are disproportionate to perceptuospatial impairment, and are sufficiently severe to hinder manual manipulation of objects and the execution of appropriate movements on walking. This problem results, not from a primary impairment in the motor system, but a failure in the translation of an intention into the appropriate motor act (apraxia).

Social graces are relatively well maintained in AD and the magnitude of the cognitive disorder is often masked by the person's normal social façade. In conversation, appropriate intonation and word emphasis and the effective use of social platitudes conveys an impression of normal communication, which contrasts with the paucity of informative speech content. People with AD may not complain of symptoms spontaneously, yet may become distressed by socially demanding situations and by test failures, indicating some maintenance of awareness.

People with AD are typically physically well in the early stages, without neurological signs. With progression of disease akinesia, rigidity and myoclonic jerking movements may emerge reflecting the gradual involvement of subcortical structures. Physical problems are nevertheless invariably overshadowed by the momentous cognitive disturbance.

Individual differences: Focal presentations of Alzheimer's disease

AD is normally associated with a cluster of symptoms, which include memory loss, perceptuospatial impairment and changes in language skills. The relative emphasis on each of these symptoms varies. Some people have a very dense amnesia with relatively mild problems in other domains. Other people have striking spatial deficits whereas their memory impairment is relatively slight. Moreover, the presentation of AD can be remarkably focal with symptoms, at least in the initial stages, occurring in a single, specific domain. This reflects a circumscribed distribution of pathological change, in one lobe or hemisphere of the brain. It has already been noted that some people with AD have a relatively selective impairment of memory, which may persist for many years before the emergence of any other symptoms, and that this selective amnesia reflects circumscribed atrophy of medial temporal lobe structures. Other people may present initially with 'visual' problems. Usually, visual symptoms reflect problems in space appreciation and are associated with parietal lobe dysfunction. The difficulty might come to light because of a series of minor car accidents, involving, for example, hitting the kerb or a parked car when driving. Such errors result from poor judgement of the spatial relationship between the driver's car and other objects. Occasionally, focal visual symptoms occur in the realm of object or face perception:

the person has difficulty recognizing objects or faces through vision even though they have no difficulty recognizing them from touch or auditory cues. A problem with object perception typically results from a difficulty forming a complete percept from perceptual elements. The person may perceive lines and edges, detect colour and may distinguish a shiny from a matt surface, but have difficulty integrating that elementary visual information into an overall perceptual configuration. The person does not perceive the complete object. People with such problems may make educated guesses about what they see on the basis of the elementary information available to them. For example, they may distinguish their nail scissors on the bathroom shelf from other items on the basis of the shiny, metallic surface. Misperceptions typically reflect the person's ability to perceive parts rather than the whole of the object. For example, a picture of a camel might be interpreted as a hill, based on perception only of the camel's hump. Perceptual problems as a dominant presenting feature of AD are relatively unusual and reflect selective posterior cortical changes.

People who present with 'visual' problems almost invariably initially attribute the problem to the eyes. They assume that they need new glasses, will go to the opticians and often seek a specialist opinion from an ophthalmologist. The problem is not at the ocular level. The problem lies at the cerebral level and reflects an impairment in the ability to process visual stimuli normally. Recognition of the nature of the problem is important to save the person multiple, fruitless consultations with eye specialists and unnecessary expenditure on spectacles, which cannot alleviate the problem.

Some people with AD present initially with language problems, particularly in word-finding and they may make sound-based errors or substitute wrong words. The language presentation of AD reflects focal degeneration affecting the left hemisphere of the brain more than the right.

Recognition that focal presentations of AD exist is important from the management perspective. Current criteria for AD (McKhann et al, 1984) specify that a probable diagnosis of AD requires the presence of memory impairment together with deficits in at least one other domain. Clearly, patients with focal presentations would not fulfil such diagnostic criteria and thus would not be eligible for new treatments for AD. Yet, ironically, it is specifically people with highly selective deficits, particularly of memory known to depend on cholinergic function, who ought theoretically to derive the most benefit from cholinergic-based pharmacological agents.

Clinical investigations in Alzheimer's disease

The electroencephalogram (EEG) shows progressive slowing of waveforms. This is a relatively non-specific finding, and therefore is helpful in supporting the diagnosis of dementia but not in the differentiation of AD from other forms of dementia. Structural brain imaging, using magnetic resonance imaging (MRI) or computed tomography (CT) shows cerebral atrophy but usually does not reveal clear regional differences in the distribution of degenerative change. Functional imaging techniques, such as positron emission tomography (PET) and single-photon emission CT (SPECT), which measure blood flow and/or cerebral perfusion, are highly informative, and typically reveal characteristic abnormalities in the temporoparietal regions. There may be extension into the frontal parts of the brain, particularly with progression of disease, but abnormalities in the anterior parts of the brain alone are exceedingly rare. PET or SPECT abnormalities reflect the pattern of clinical symptoms. People with dominant problems in memory and word-finding show predominant changes in the temporal lobes, whereas spatial problems are associated with parietal lobe abnormalities. Normally, the abnormalities on functional imaging are bilateral and relatively symmetrical, affecting the left and right temporoparietal regions equally. However, focal presentations of AD may be associated with asymmetric findings. People presenting with language problems may show more left-sided change and those presenting with spatial difficulties more right-sided change.

Pathology

Atrophy is widespread, but is most intense in the temporoparietal and medial temporal regions. The characteristic histological appearances are of an initial deposition of β-A4 amyloid, followed by senile plaques consisting of degenerating neuronal processes and finally the development of intraneuronal neurofibrillary tangles, leading to the death of large cortical neurons. Amyloid may also be deposited in cortical blood vessels, also known as amyloid angiopathy.

Genetics

AD most often occurs sporadically, without an obvious familial link. However, in a proportion of people the illness is clearly familial, affecting individuals in successive generations in a dominant inheritance fashion. Genetic mutations have been identified on chromosomes 1, 14 and 21, demonstrating that familial AD is not homogeneous. Chromosome 14 mutations have been particularly associated with very young onset AD, beginning often in the forties. There is now increasing evidence that even in people in whom the disease is not obviously familial there may be genetic influences that have the effect of predisposing (rather than causing) an individual to develop AD. One of these is apolipoprotein E (Apo E). As yet, established genetic factors that increase susceptibility to AD do not account for the entire spectrum of AD. In many people with AD, including those with young onset disease, the underlying contributions to the disease remain unknown.

Down's syndrome

Many people with the learning disorder Down's syndrome (DS) develop an Alzheimer-type dementia during their life. The prevalence increases with advancing age, with only 1% or 2% of people being affected in their 30s, and up to 75% after the age of 50. There is no evidence to suggest that people with more severe forms of DS are more vulnerable to dementia than those with less severe forms. DS relates to the effects of trisomy of chromosome 21. This chromosome contains the gene coding for amyloid precursor protein (APP), and it is a mutation in this gene that is responsible for some cases of early onset AD. In DS there is increasing deposition over time of diffuse amyloid in the brain, followed progressively by the formation of neuritic plaques, neurofibrillary tangles, neuronal loss and cerebral atrophy, namely, development of the pathological changes of AD. The dementia that follows is that of AD, characterized by problems in memory, visuospatial function, praxis and language.

The detection of the emergence of dementia in people with DS is not straightforward, being complicated by the presence of the pre-existing learning disorder. It is often difficult to disentangle newly acquired cognitive impairments from long-standing cognitive difficulties related to the developmental disorder. Behavioural disorders heralding the onset of dementia may be difficult to separate from those attributable to depression, hypothyroidism, sensory deprivation or the effects of life events. Moreover, little is known of the impact on brain imaging of an acquired cerebral degeneration on a congenitally compromised brain, so that brain imaging findings may be difficult to interpret. The identification of dementia in DS is often highly dependent on the careful observations of caregivers who have known individuals for a prolonged period of time and are able to provide an account of cognitive and functional decline.

Frontotemporal dementia
Frontotemporal dementia (FTD) (Gustafson et al, 1987; Neary et al, 1988; Snowden et al, 1996) is the most common form of primary degenerative dementia after AD that affects people in middle age, accounting for at least one in eight cases of dementia before age 65, making it one of the more common types of dementia affecting younger people. Frontotemporal dementia begins most commonly between the ages of 45 and 65. However, it can occur in both older and younger individuals, the youngest onset in our own experience being 21 years. The average duration of illness is 8 years, although there is marked variation with a range from 2 to 20 years. The disorder occurs with roughly equal frequency in men and women, in contrast to AD, which is more prevalent in women. It is a more strongly familial disorder than AD, a family history of a similar disorder in a first degree relative being present in up to 50% of cases.

The disorder occurs in all parts of the world. However, as in other strongly familial disorders there may be regional variations in prevalence reflecting the presence in some regions of familial clusters. No environmental determinants have hitherto been detected.

Clinical characteristics of frontotemporal dementia

FTD is clinically distinct from AD. Table 2.2 lists the main differentiating features. It is characterized by profound alteration in a person's personality and social conduct. Whereas the earliest symptoms in AD are cognitive, those in FTD are behavioural and affective. Symptoms include poor judgement, neglect of occupational and domestic responsibilities, socially inappropriate behaviour, lack of concern, self-centredness and a lack of sympathy or empathy for others. The presence of the disorder may come to light in an occupational setting. For example, an electrician was noted by his employers to be acting the fool wearing a monkey's mask and bucket on his head, while working at great height. He was oblivious of the danger to himself or fellow workmates. Alternatively, symptoms may come to light in a social setting. For example, one individual caused considerable distress by recounting dirty jokes with great hilarity while attending a funeral. Another appeared unmoved by the death of a close and beloved relative and remarked callously that it was 'one less present to buy at Christmas'. In each case the behavioural symptom was regarded by relatives as totally out of character.

Alterations in mood are invariable in FTD and strongly differentiate FTD from other forms of dementia, particularly AD. FTD patients are typically reported by their relatives to show a general reduction in their display of emotion. They no longer show appropriate signs of happiness, sadness, anger, fear, surprise or disgust. Moreover, they do not show social emotions of embarrassment or sympathy. Such a pervasive loss of emotion is much less commonly reported in other forms of dementia. Another prominent behavioural characteristic in FTD is alteration in eating habits. Eating changes in FTD include excessive, indiscriminate eating, food cramming, seeking out food, and stealing food from the plates of others. Food fads and an altered preference

Table 2.2 Comparison of clinical features in Alzheimer's disease (AD) and frontotemporal dementia (FTD)

	AD	FTD
Presenting features	Cognitive change	Behavioural/character change
Cognitive characteristics	Memory impairment Spatial disorientation Language disorder	Concreteness of thought Impaired problem-solving Impaired set-shifting/ perseveration
Neurological signs	Akinesia, rigidity, myoclonus	Primitive reflexes Late akinesia and rigidity
Social interaction	Preserved social skills	Socially inappropriate
Affect	Anxious, concerned	Blunted, fatuous, unconcerned
EEG	Slow waves	Normal
Structural imaging	Generalized atrophy	Atrophy, may show frontal emphasis
Functional imaging	Posterior cerebral abnormality	Anterior cerebral abnormality

for sweet foods are common. Such changes are rare in other forms of dementia. Another prominent and discriminating characteristic of FTD is the presence of repetitive, stereotyped behaviours. These may constitute simple mannerisms, such as repetitive humming, grunting, foot tapping or hand rubbing, or more complex routines, such as clapping out the same rhythm repetitively, singing the same song, dancing the same dance or saying the same phrase. In some instances, they constitute lengthy and elaborate behavioural rituals. For example, one individual would empty all the clothes from her wardrobe each morning and pile them on to a wheelchair, which she would push from her bedroom to the hospital dayroom. At an appointed time each afternoon she would push the wheelchair back to her bedroom and return her clothes to their correct position in the wardrobe. Wandering is a common feature, which often has a repetitive quality, involving pacing a fixed route. Some people with FTD exhibit stimulus-bound behaviour, in which the person grasps and uses objects in their visual field, despite the contextual inappropriateness. Thus, a person in the home of a neighbour might pick up the neighbour's comb and begin combing his or her own hair. This is known as utilization behaviour and it can have a markedly repetitive quality. A person may persist in a previously appropriate activity when it is no longer appropriate, such as carrying on drinking from an empty cup.

Cognitive changes are predominantly in the realm of frontal executive functions. People with FTD show impairments in attention, problem-solving, organizational and sequencing abilities. They are concrete in their thinking and show difficulty shifting mental set. Perseverative responses are common. Test performance is often characterized by poor persistence on tasks, reduced mental effort, and economical and cursory responses. Primary perceptual and spatial skills remain well preserved. People with FTD may remain oriented in their surroundings, and may be able to localize and align objects even in very late stage disease. Nevertheless, performance on formal tests of these functions may be compromised secondarily by inattention, inefficient retrieval strategies, poor organization, poor mental application and effort, lack of self-monitoring and lack of concern for accuracy.

Speech output in FTD is economical and concrete, and verbatim copying of what is said by others (echolalia) and repetition of their own responses (perseveration) may occur. There may be stereotyped repetition of a word, phrase or complete theme. Mutism invariably ensues late in the disease.

As in AD, people with FTD are generally physically well and the behavioural abnormalities far outweigh physical symptoms. Neurological signs are typically absent early in the disease or limited to the presence of primitive reflexes, such as automatic grasping when the palm of the outstretched hand is stroked. With disease progression parkinsonian signs of akinesia and rigidity develop and may be marked in some people. Moreover, in a minority of people, FTD occurs in association with the neurological signs of motor neuron disease (MND). In these people the duration of illness is dramatically shortened to 2 or 3 years as a consequence of the co-occurrence of MND.

Behavioural subtypes of frontotemporal dementia

Behavioural changes in people with FTD can take different forms, depending on the parts of the frontotemporal lobes most affected by the disease. People with atrophy confined to the orbitomedial frontal lobes and temporal poles are disinhibited, fatuous, distractible and socially inappropriate. They may be impulsive, restless and purposelessly overactive. People with widespread frontal lobe atrophy extending into the dorsolateral parts of the frontal lobes show a picture of underactivity. They are bland, apathetic, lacking in volition and mental effort, mentally inflexible and perseverative. Repetitive, stereotyped behaviours may be associated with both behavioural types. However, in some people with FTD in whom there is marked striatotemporal involvement, ritualistic behaviours may be the dominant feature. These are often of the superstitious type, such as avoiding walking on cracks in the pavement, and have a compulsive quality, such as tapping each of the four walls three times on entering a room.

Clinical investigations in frontotemporal dementia

The EEG is invariably normal. This is important diagnostically because most other forms of dementia are associated with an abnormal EEG. Structural brain imaging shows cerebral atrophy, the preferential atrophy of the frontal and anterior temporal lobes typically being

22

demonstrable on MRI. Functional imaging techniques such as SPECT (which provides information about blood flow and perfusion via a gamma camera) reveal characteristic abnormalities in the anterior cerebral hemispheres. These are bilateral, but may be asymmetric, with greater involvement of one hemisphere than the other.

Pathology

Postmortem pathological examination of the brain reveals bilateral atrophy of the frontal and anterior temporal lobes and degeneration of the striatum. Histological findings are of three main types (Lund and Manchester groups, 1994). The most common (microvacuolar-type), accounting for about 60% of cases, is characterized by loss of large cortical nerve cells with a sponge-like (spongiform) appearance and there are no distinctive changes (swellings or inclusions) within remaining nerve cells. A second histological pattern accounting for approximately 25% is characterized by a loss of large cortical nerve cells with widespread and abundant gliosis but minimal or no spongiform change. This has been referred to as Pick-type histology. Swollen neurons or inclusions within the cells are present in most cases. The two differing microscopic appearances share a similar distribution within the frontal and temporal cortex. In about 15% of cases, clinical features of FTD+MND are present during life, usually with a pathological appearance of the first variant, or very rarely a Pick-type pathology is combined with those of MND. It is because the histopathological characteristics underlying FTD vary that the clinical term FTD is favoured over the eponymous, pathologically-based label 'Pick's disease'.

Genetics

FTD is a more strongly familial disorder than AD, and a family history of the same disease is present in about 40% of cases. Mutations in the tau gene on chromosome 17 have been identified in some families (Hutton et al, 1998). However, like AD, there is not a single genetic cause. In non-familial cases factors underlying development of the disease are unknown.

23

Clinical syndromes related to frontotemporal dementia

The behavioural disorder of FTD is the most common of a variety of clinical syndromes associated with focal degeneration of the anterior parts of the brain and that share the same underlying non-Alzheimer histological characteristics (Snowden et al, 1996; Neary et al, 1998). This group of conditions is also sometimes known as the 'lobar atrophies'. The clinical syndrome is determined by the distribution of pathology within the brain (Figure 2.2). As noted above, FTD is associated with bilateral atrophy of the frontal and anterior temporal lobes. Asymmetrical involvement predominantly of the left dominant anterior hemisphere leads to the syndrome of *progressive non-fluent aphasia*. Predominant involvement of the inferior and middle gyri of both temporal lobes leads to a syndrome of fluent aphasia with associative visual agnosia, known as *semantic dementia*. Focal degeneration of the frontoparietal regions is associated with the syndrome of *progressive apraxia*. The demographic characteristics are similar to those of FTD. Each of these syndromes may be familial or occur sporadically and each is usually (although not always) associated with onset before the age of 65 years. The disorder occurs in the context of physical well-being. As in FTD the EEG is normal. Findings on neuroimaging reflect the distribution of pathological change.

Progressive non-fluent aphasia

In this form of lobar degeneration (Snowden et al, 1996), a progressive decline in language occurs in the relative absence of other cognitive deficits, and because of the selectivity of the disorder affected individuals may maintain a high level of functional independence. Speech is non-fluent, effortful and lacking in prosody. Word retrieval difficulties are prominent and there are typically, although not invariably, sound-based (phonemic paraphasic) errors. The ability to repeat, to produce overlearnt series, such as the days of the week, to read aloud, write and spell, are also affected, but spoken and written comprehension at least at the single word level are relatively preserved. Behavioural change akin to that of FTD may develop late in the disease, reflecting a spread of pathology to both frontotemporal lobes.

Semantic dementia

This disorder (Snowden et al, 1989, 1996) is characterized by a loss of meaning. The earliest symptom is often in the realm of language, and reflects a breakdown in understanding of word meaning. The person has difficulty in naming, makes word errors that are semantically related to the correct word (e.g. 'dog' for rabbit) and shows impaired understanding of nominal terms, as demonstrated by comments such as 'rabbit, what's a rabbit? I don't know what that is'. The breakdown in semantics is not confined to word meaning but progressively affects all sensory domains. Thus, affected individuals have difficulty recognizing familiar faces. They may no longer appreciate the meaning of objects, non-verbal environmental sounds such as the ringing of a doorbell, or water running from a tap. Non-semantic aspects of cognitive function are well preserved. Spontaneous speech is fluent, effortless and grammatically correct, and may at least in the initial stages appear superficially normal. However, it become progressively empty of content and the person relies increasingly on stock phrases and uses terms over-inclusively. The ability to repeat, read aloud and write to dictation regularly spelt words is essentially intact, reflecting preservation of phonological and articulatory skills. Difficulties in recognizing the significance of objects and the identity of faces occurs despite a preserved ability to copy accurately and match objects and faces. That is, the person perceives the object or face normally. The problem is in attributing a meaning to the normal percept. In contrast to AD, visuospatial skills are invariably normal, so that the person has no difficulty negotiating their environment, in orienting clothing when dressing and localizing objects. Moreover, day-to-day memorizing is well preserved, contrasting with the striking loss of semantic knowledge. Behavioural alterations occur, which often have a compulsive quality. The person clockwatches, adheres to a fixed routine, carrying out the same activities at an identical time each day, and may be preoccupied by a very limited set of pursuits, neglecting other responsibilities. Prominent temporal lobe atrophy is invariably detected by MRI. SPECT shows reduced uptake of tracer in anterior regions. The EEG is normal.

Progressive apraxia

This disorder (Dick et al, 1989) is characterized by a selective loss of the ability to carry out skilled actions. The first symptoms are often difficulty in carrying out actions involving fine movements such as writing or drawing. Bimanual actions, such as using a knife and fork or tying shoelaces, may be particularly difficult. Progressively, the apraxia affects lower limb, buccofacial and whole body movements so the person becomes totally dependent on others for activities of daily living. The clinical syndrome of progressive apraxia differs from that of the corticosubcortical disorder of corticobasal degeneration (discussed later) principally on the basis of the absence of subcortical signs of parkinsonism and slowing in mentation, and the symmetrical nature of the apraxia.

Lobar degeneration and motor neurone disease

The clinical syndromes of frontotemporal lobar degeneration are complicated in a minority of cases by the development of the amyotrophic form of MND. Typically, the neurological symptoms and signs commence after the development of the dementia and lead to death within three years from respiratory complications. Electrophysiological studies demonstrate widespread damage in the form of denervation of muscles.

Alcoholic dementia

Alcohol abuse can damage both limbic structures and the frontal lobes, resulting in memory and/or frontal executive impairments. The amnesic syndrome usually arises following an acute neurological crisis (Wernicke's encephalopathy) (Victor et al, 1971). The patient sinks into stupor or coma, develops ocular paralyses, irregularly-sized pupils and gait disturbance (ataxia). Individuals who survive may be left with a profound and yet relatively circumscribed amnesia (Korsakoff's amnesia or Wernicke-Korsakoff syndrome). Such individuals may be relatively free from frontal (executive) impairments. Moreover, unlike people with AD, in whom memory loss is progressive, the amnesia is static or may improve to some degree following a period of abstinence. However, a proportion of chronic alcohol abusers who neglect their diet, present with a progressive dementing syndrome in which there are features of both amnesia and frontal lobe disturbance. In such individuals there is a progressive decline in mental function, so that the disorder needs to be distinguished from degenerative conditions such as AD and frontotemporal dementia. CT and MRI evidence of cerebral atrophy is seen in the majority of individuals with both the acute and chronic alcoholic syndromes.

Subcortical dementias

Several diseases that can give rise to dementia predominantly affect subcortical structures. These include the degenerative disorders of subcortical grey matter: progressive supranuclear palsy, Parkinson's disease and Huntington's disease, as well as subcortical white matter disorders such as vascular disease (subcortical arteriosclerotic dementia), repeated head trauma (boxer's encephalopathy), multiple sclerosis and the rare late onset leukodystrophies (discussed later). Diseases of the subcortex share commonalities with respect to the pattern of mental change and have been referred to as the 'subcortical dementias' (Cummings, 1990). They differ from cortical dementias both in terms of the form of the dementia and the presence of physical abnormalities. Cortical dementias, such as AD and FTD, are associated with severe and incapacitating mental changes and relatively mild physical changes. By contrast, in subcortical disorders the reverse is the case. The neuropsychological deficits are usually overshadowed by profound and characteristic neurological symptoms and signs.

Progressive supranuclear palsy

Progressive supranuclear palsy (PSP) is a degenerative neurological disorder characterized by paralysis of eye movements, parkinsonian features and dementia. It is more common in males and is typically sporadic. It usually begins around the sixth decade of life and the total

27

disease course is between 4 and 7 years. The earliest symptoms are typically physical: sufferers may complain of unsteadiness or abrupt falls. However, mental symptoms are also present. PSP represents the prototypical subcortical dementia. Affected individuals are slowed down in their thinking and show reduced mental flexibility. They have difficulty switching 'mental set' from one task to another or one response mode to another, so that responses are frequently perseverative. Memory is inefficient and there is difficulty in the active retrieval of information, but people with PSP are not amnesic in the same way as a person with AD. Cognitive assessment reveals greatest difficulty on tests sensitive to frontal lobe function that require organization, planning and sequencing and active mental manipulation of information. People with PSP do not make specific linguistic errors in speech: there is simply an economy of output. They show good visual perceptual and spatial skills. Typically, they do not show the gross personality alteration and breakdown in social awareness seen in frontal cortical disease. Structural brain imaging may be normal or show non-specific cerebral atrophy. Functional imaging (SPECT) typically shows abnormalities in the anterior hemispheres.

Parkinson's disease
Parkinson's disease (PD) is typically thought of as a movement rather than cognitive disorder and it is certainly the characteristic akinesia, rigidity and tremor that dominate the clinical picture. Nevertheless, some cognitive changes may be present akin to those seen in PSP, with slowing of mental function, reduced mental flexibility and inefficient retrieval of information. The severity of the mental changes varies in degree and in only a proportion of people may lead to significant management problems. The emergence of clear cortical cognitive features in addition to the subcortical pattern mental change suggests a diagnosis of Lewy body dementia, to be discussed later.

Huntington's disease
Huntington's disease (HD) is a genetic disorder with an autosomal dominant mode of inheritance (Harper et al, 2002). Onset occurs on

average between the ages of 40 and 45, but there is wide variation. Very rarely, onset may occur in childhood. Equally rarely, it may develop in people over the age of 70. The duration of illness is typically between 15 and 20 years, although both shorter and longer durations have been reported. HD is distinguished clinically by its characteristic involuntary movements. The identification in 1993 of the genetic mutation responsible for HD on chromosome 4 means that a genetic test for the disorder is now possible, so that a definitive diagnosis can be made in life.

Although the involuntary movements are the most visible sign of HD it is the accompanying behavioural and cognitive changes that present the greatest challenge for management. The cognitive changes are largely similar in kind to those of other forms of subcortical dementia (slowing of mentation, mental inflexibility and inefficient memorizing), although they are often more pronounced than in PSP or PD. Behavioural changes include reduced initiative, mental intransigence, self-centredness and a loss of sympathy and empathy for others, irritability and aggression.

Vascular dementia: Subcortical arteriosclerotic type

When vascular lesions predominantly affect the subcortical white matter, a characteristic subcortical syndrome (subcortical arteriosclerotic dementia) emerges which is similar to that of subcortical degenerative disease. Affected individuals are mentally (as well as physically) slowed, they show impaired mental flexibility and inefficient generative and retrieval skills. Vascular causes of subcortical dementia need to be distinguished from degenerative causes. A common preconception is that, whereas degenerative forms of dementia are associated with an insidious onset and gradually progressive course, vascular dementia has an acute onset and stepwise progression. Although this is true for cortical vascular disease, it is not so of subcortical arteriosclerotic dementia. Like degenerative dementias the disorder progresses gradually. Differentiation from degenerative dementias is made largely on the clinical history, neurological signs and presence of risk factors for cerebrovascular disease.

CADASIL

Cerebral autosomal dominant arteriopathy with subcortical infarcts and leukoencephalopathy (CADASIL) is a familial form of subcortical vascular disease, which may present with migraine, transient ischaemic attacks or stroke. However, some people present with a chronic, progressive subcortical dementia without ictal events. MRI of the brain reveals multifocal subcortical infarcts and leukoaraiosis, most marked in the temporal lobes and also involving the corpus collosum. Diagnosis is by skin biopsy to detect small vessel disease and DNA analysis to detect mutations of the 'notch' gene on chromosome 19.

Multiple sclerosis

Multiple sclerosis is a disorder that affects white matter tracts within the central nervous system and is most common in young adults. Although the disorder is typically associated with a relapsing–remitting course and physical symptomatology, mental changes may also occur and very occasionally dementia is the presenting symptom. Slowing of mental function and apathy reflect the predominantly frontal lobe distribution of the subcortical lesions. MRI of the brain reveals asymmetrical white matter hyperintense lesions especially anteriorly, around the ventricles and in the corpus collosum. Cerebrospinal fluid (CSF) examination reveals a characteristic increase of protein content with a distinct appearance, known as oligoclonal bands.

Late onset leukodystrophies

The leukodystrophies are inborn errors of metabolism, manifesting normally in childhood, but occasionally presenting in young adults. Two diseases are chiefly responsible, metachromatic leukodystrophy (a lysosomal disorder) and adrenoleukodystrophy (a peroxisomal disorder). The mode of inheritance is autosomal recessive and X-linked recessive, respectively. Clinically, corticospinal symptoms and signs of weakness and spasticity together with ataxia are followed by progressive dementia, epilepsy and myoclonus. A peripheral neuropathy may coexist. MRI of the brain reveals confluent and symmetrical attenuation of cerebral white matter with lesser involvement of the cerebral cortex. Diagnosis is biochemical. In metachromatic leukodystrophy assays of aryl sulphatase A in white blood cells reveals enzyme deficiency. In adrenoleukodystrophy very long chain fatty acids are raised in plasma and fibroblasts.

Human immunodeficiency virus dementia

Dementia occurs in a proportion of people with human immunodeficiency virus (HIV) infection. Prevalence estimates suggest that between 7% and 10% of people with symptomatic HIV disease have dementia, and these figures rise to between 15% and 20% for people with advanced HIV disease. Cognitive impairment conforms to a subcortical picture. The salient features are mental slowing, poor concentration and inefficient memory. Cognitive changes are often accompanied by alterations in behaviour, and these strongly suggest involvement of the subcortico–frontocortical circuitry. Some individuals become inert, apathetic and withdrawn, lacking in motivation and drive. Others show a more overactive, disinhibited profile, akin to hypomania. In keeping with the clinical picture, functional imaging using PET has demonstrated regional metabolic changes in prefrontal areas and the basal ganglia. People with HIV dementia typically also show physical impairments. These include weakness, clumsiness and ataxia, and ultimately paralysis and incontinence.

The primary histological brain changes in HIV dementia are of inflammatory foci of microglia, macrophages and multinucleated giant cells leading to myelin loss, reactive astrocytosis and neuronal loss. The white matter bears the brunt of the damage (HIV leukoencephalopathy) with less frequent primary involvement of grey matter in the basal ganglia and cerebral cortex (poliodystrophy) or blood vessels (cerebral vasculitis).

Corticosubcortical encephalopathy

Two degenerative disorders show features of both cortical and subcortical syndromes determined by the spread of pathology to both structures. In Lewy body disease the distribution of pathology is symmetrical whereas in corticobasal degeneration it is highly asymmetrical. Vascular disease may also affect both cortex and subcortex.

Dementia with Lewy bodies

Dementia with Lewy bodies (DLB) (McKeith et al, 1996) is a disorder that more commonly affects the elderly, although it can occur in younger people. It is typically sporadic. Mental changes develop before or after parkinsonian symptoms and signs of akinesia, rigidity and tremor that are responsive to the administration of the drug L-dopa. Changes in the cerebral cortex give rise to cortical symptoms, which bear similarities to those of AD. Nevertheless, there are features that clearly distinguish the two conditions. A dominant feature of DLB is a fluctuating mental state, so that the person may appear lucid at times but incoherent and confused at others. Such fluctuations, which are presumably due to simultaneous disorder of cortex and subcortex, are highly diagnostic, since they are not characteristic of the cortical or subcortical encephalopathies. When 'confusion' does occur in these latter disorders it usually relates to systemic complications, drug toxicity, anaesthesia or the relative sensory deprivation of night-time or unfamiliar surroundings. A second common characteristic of DLB is the presence of visual illusions and hallucinations. Hallucinations are formed and are typically of animals or people. They do not usually cause distress to the person. Another striking feature of DLB, which is likely to relate to fluctuating attention, is the presence of intrusion errors, which may be elicited by extraneous objects in the visual environment. For example, in the process of relating the activities of the previous day a person with DLB might incorporate irrelevant words from a notice on the wall on which his/her gaze happens to fall (e.g. 'yesterday, we went to the Fire Exit'). Such errors are not a notable feature of AD.

The EEG in DLB characteristically reveals severe slowing of waveforms and sometimes periodic wavecomplexes. CT reveals cerebral atrophy. SPECT reveals reductions of uptake in the cerebral cortex especially in the posterior hemispheres as in AD.

Corticobasal degeneration

In corticobasal degeneration (Gibb et al, 1989; Riley et al, 1990) a cortical syndrome of apraxia is superimposed upon a subcortical form of dementia. The disorder most often begins in middle life and progresses over about 5 years. The presenting symptom is typically of difficulty in the use of one or other upper limb, although the apraxia typically progresses to involve both upper limbs, as well as the mouth (buccofacial), lower limb and whole body movements. The limbs progressively lose all executive functions and may develop autonomous movements (sometimes called 'alien limb'). The person is unable to carry out manual tasks and so becomes totally dependent on others for activities of daily living. The apraxia is ideomotor rather than conceptual in type. That is, the person retains knowledge of the nature of the action that he/she is trying to execute, but is unable to implement the action effectively. Understandably, this leads to feelings of profound frustration and distress. Progressively there are difficulties with speech, so that communication is compromised, further increasing the person's isolation and potential distress. Although apraxia is the prominent cortical feature, additional features of parietal lobe disease, namely, visuospatial deficits, may also emerge. Subcortical features of mental slowing, inflexibility and perseveration are also present.

Neurological signs are of basal ganglia disorder. Asymmetrical akinesia and rigidity affect predominantly the upper limbs, which are also the site of tremor, dystonic movements and myoclonus. EEG changes are of non-specific asymmetrical slow waves. CT reveals cerebral atrophy. Functional imaging (PET and SPECT) reveals asymmetrical abnormalities of the basal ganglia and associated frontoparietal cortex.

Vascular dementia

Recurrent completed strokes lead to an accumulated neurological and psychological deficit, resembling a dementia syndrome. As the disorder is associated with discrete, acute stroke-like events, each associated with a stepwise decline in function, and there is typically evidence of multiple infarctions or haemorrhages on brain imaging, this form of vascular dementia is not likely to lead to diagnostic confusion. In a proportion of patients, however, vascular events occur both in the cortex and the subcortex, but without evident historical stroke-like events. The clinical picture of multiple (cortical and subcortical) infarct dementia may superficially resemble AD. CT, MRI and functional brain imaging reveals asymmetrically distributed focal lesions in the cerebral hemispheres.

Multifocal encephalopathy

Creutzfeldt–Jakob disease

Creutzfeldt–Jakob disease (Matthews, 1985) is a rapidly progressive brain disorder, which tends to affect people in middle life and is often terminal within 6 months of onset. Longer survival may occur in familial disease forms such as Gerstmann–Straussler–Sheinker syndrome.

The presenting symptoms can differ widely. Some people present with neurological symptoms such as unsteadiness, sensory motor deficits, myoclonus and epileptic seizures. Other people present with focal cortical symptoms such as visual failure or language disorder. Involvement of the deep structures, such as the thalamus, may lead to progressive somnolence (fatal insomnia). In some people, initial symptoms are relatively non-specific and include difficulties in concentration, lethargy and malaise. Despite the apparent heterogeneity of presenting symptoms, there are nevertheless common characteristics, rarely seen in other encephalopathies. Commonly, there are fluctuations in the person's responsiveness. Periods of unresponsiveness, in which the person is immobile with a fixed gaze intervene between periods of appropriate responsiveness and interaction, during which the person may comment on events occurring during their non-responsive states, indicating that they are conscious and able to process and assimilate information effectively. Periods of unresponsiveness vary in duration. They may initially be fleeting, lasting only seconds, but they become progressively prolonged over the course of the disorder leading ultimately to a state of akinetic mutism. As in DLB, which affects both cortex and subcortex, intrusion errors and response perseverations are common in CJD.

The severe neurological and psychological disorder is reflected in the grossly disturbed EEG in which there is profound slowing of waveforms and characteristic periodic triphasic wavecomplexes emerge. CT is either normal or reveals non-specific cerebral atrophy. SPECT imaging reveals a patchy reduction of uptake of tracer in the cerebral cortex.

New variant Creutzfeldt–Jakob disease (vCJD)

This form of CJD, first reported in 1996 (Will et al, 1996, 2000) is attributed to infection with the agent causing bovine spongiform encephalopathy (BSE). Unlike classical CJD, which affects people in middle age, vCJD commonly affects younger people, the average age of onset being 26 years. The average duration of illness is about 13 months. The earliest symptoms are usually psychiatric, and include depression, withdrawal, aggression and irritability, anxiety and fear, hallucinations and delusions. Cognitive changes frequently take the form of a subcortical dementia, with mental slowing and inefficient memorizing, although as expected in a multifocal disorder cortical symptoms may also be present.

Differential diagnosis of dementias

Cortical, subcortical, corticosubcortical and multifocal encephalopathies differ with respect to the relative prominence of associated mental and physical changes in the evolution of disease (Table 2.3).

Table 2.3 Patterns of cognitive and neurological disorder in different forms of dementia

Part of brain most affected	Prototypical disorder	Cognitive disorder	Physical disorder
Anterior cortex	FTD	Severe, specific	Mild, occurs late
Posterior/medial cortex	AD	Severe, specific	Mild, occurs late
Subcortex	PSP	Mild, specific	Moderate, occurs early
Cortex + subcortex	DLB	Fluctuating	Moderate, occurs early
Multifocal	CJD	Severe, non-specific	Severe, diffuse

FTD, frontotemporal dementia; AD, Alzheimer's disease; PSP, progressive supranuclear palsy; DLB, dementia with Lewy bodies; CJD, Creutzfeldt–Jakob disease

Cortical encephalopathies are characterized by profound mental changes in the relative absence of early neurological signs, whereas subcortical encephalopathies are associated with striking physical signs while mental changes may be of relatively lesser significance and tend to emerge later in the disease. In corticosubcortical and multifocal encephalopathies physical symptoms and signs emerge along with the psychological disturbance.

The EEG is also of diagnostic significance. In AD, the standard EEG often shows mild slowing of waveforms in the moderately advanced stages of the disease. The clinical syndromes associated with frontotemporal lobar degeneration are unique in that a normal record is preserved until the latest stages of the disease. Gross slowing of waveforms and periodic wavecomplexes are characteristic of the subacute spongiform encephalopathies and also of cortical Lewy body disease. Whereas CT is useful in delineating structural changes, such as the presence of vascular diseases or hydrocephalus, it is less useful in differential diagnosis in neurodegenerative disorders as scans may be normal or reveal non-specific cerebral atrophy. However, high resolution MRI may be useful in highlighting prominent areas of atrophy, complementing the clinical and SPECT findings. SPECT imaging demonstrates functional change in the brain, which is of high diagnostic value in the neurodegenerative disorders, because the abnormalities on imaging closely reflect the topographical distribution of pathology within the cerebrum. The radioactive tracer crosses the blood–brain barrier and is taken up by cerebral tissue reflecting cerebral blood flow and perfusion, and hence regional metabolic function. In frontotemporal dementia the characteristic abnormality in the frontotemporal lobes contrasts strikingly with the bilateral parietal defects seen in AD. An asymmetrical dominant hemispheric defect characterizes progressive non-fluent aphasia, whereas predominantly bitemporal defects underlie semantic dementia. Subcortical disorders, such as PSP, display an anterior cerebral defect which is less severe than in lobar atrophy. An asymmetrical frontoparietal defect is seen in corticobasal degeneration.

Differentiation from extrinsic encephalopathies

Neurosurgical conditions, which lead to mechanical compression of the brain and increased space occupation within the cranium, can lead to mental changes that mimic those of intrinsic brain disease. The most common syndrome results from a space-occupying and expanding lesion within or on the surface of the brain such as a neoplasm, abscess or haematoma. Here, a focal and unilateral neuropsychological syndrome, such as aphasia and right hemiparesis, occurs which is related to the specific site of the lesion in the cerebral cortex or subcortex. These cognitive features are associated with symptoms and signs of raised intracranial pressure, namely, headache and papilloedema and progressive confusion and obtundation, and it is these latter features that alert the physician to the diagnosis.

The second extrinsic cortical syndrome is that of hydrocephalus in which, due to obstruction of the flow and absorption of CSF, the cerebral ventricles expand under the increased pressure of the CSF. A characteristic syndrome emerges in which bilateral neurological signs reflect the progressive change to the subcortical white matter and nuclei, especially those immediately adjacent to the ventricles. The gait is characteristically slow, shuffling and wide-based with the feet seemingly rooted to the ground. There is pyramidal tract weakness and spasticity of the lower limbs often with akinesia and rigidity. The upper limbs are less affected, although clumsy and incoordinate, and speech is slow, slurred and indistinct. Mental function is slowed and inefficient, with response perseverations. Concentration and memory become progressively impaired but cortical functions are unaffected, so that aphasia, agnosia, apraxia and spatial disorientation are absent. This syndrome shares commonalities with the 'subcortical dementia' described above. In the case of obstructive hydrocephalus usually due to a tumour, progress is rapid and confusion, obtundation and coma occur early, so that the diagnosis is not in doubt. However, in the case of 'communicating' hydrocephalus due to impaired CSF absorption the cause is more chronic, consciousness is disrupted later and therefore the differential diagnosis from neurodegenerative and vascular forms of dementia can be more difficult and requires both structural and functional imaging and physiological studies of the CSF pathways.

Differentiation from metabolic encephalopathies

Another important group of disorders of general medical significance, which must be distinguished from progressive dementia syndromes, are those arising when systemic disorders attack a potentially intact nervous system. Cerebral impairment fluctuates in degree as a function of the severity of the general medical disorder, and constitutes a distinct clinical syndrome, referred to as a 'confusional state', intermediate between full arousal and unresponsive coma. The reduced level of arousal leads secondarily to reduced cognitive efficiency. Mental and physical tasks are carried out more slowly, and the ability to sustain attention and attend selectively in the face of distraction is severely compromised. Drowsiness and sleepiness may be evident. Rapid fluctuations of alertness occur. Before coma supervenes behaviour may be overactive and purposeless (delirium). Language is not frankly dysphasic insofar as grammatical and phonemic paraphasic errors are absent, but affected individuals are unable to maintain a coherent train of thought so that content of speech is irrelevant and often incomprehensible. Written expressions are typically even more incoherent than spoken utterances, and may contain perseverations of words and individual pencil strokes. Naming errors occur, with verbal substitutions and perseverations, although these are inconsistent over repeated trials. Misperception leads to illusions and hallucinations, often of a fearful aspect. Patients have difficulty carrying out all tasks requiring organizational skills. Constructional tasks, such as copying drawings, and spatial tasks, such as maze-trailing are failed. There is disorientation, particularly for time, but often also for place, but never for personal identity. The purposeful regulation of behaviour becomes impossible leading to erratic responses and motiveless wandering. Neurological signs frequently accompany metabolic encephalopathy and include postural tremor, asterixis (a flapping movement of the outstretched hands) and myoclonus. The EEG typically reveals diffuse slow wave large amplitude waveforms. Metabolic encephalopathy may be produced by a variety of systemic diseases, including hepatic, renal and cardiorespiratory encephalopathies, deficiency states such as vitamin B_{12} deficiency, endocrine disorders, such as hypoglycaemia and hypothyroidism, and disorders of electrolyte imbalance, such as hyponatraemia, and hypocalcaemia. In addition to the characteristic neuropsychological syndrome there is evidence of systemic disease on clinical examination and haematological, biochemical and endocrine investigation.

Metabolic encephalopathy accounts for a very small proportion of the chronic syndromes typically encountered by specialists in dementia. Nevertheless, recognition of its features is essential so that it can be accurately distinguished from dementia due to progressive intrinsic brain disease. The clinical differentiation is of high therapeutic import as the metabolic encephalopathies are essentially treatable. Diagnosis and treatment of systemic disease, especially in the early stages, can lead to a complete resolution of the metabolic encephalopathy.

Diagnostic criteria for degenerative diseases such as AD typically cite confusional states as an exclusion criterion. Yet, people with AD and other degenerative dementias are not immune from the coincidental development of metabolic encephalopathies. Indeed, they may be more susceptible than other people because they have less cerebral reserve. The development of fluctuations in arousal and especially nocturnal confusion in people with dementia should alert carers to the possibility of systemic complications such as drug intoxication or infection.

Conclusion

Dementia is a generic term embracing a number of neuropsychological syndromes associated with a wide variety of brain diseases. Dementia is not a generalized and uniform impairment of mental function. Younger people with dementia have specific, identifiable clusters of difficulties that vary from one person to another and more particularly, from one disease to another. The pattern of mental change reflects the parts of the brain most affected by the disease process. Understanding the specific symptoms associated with different disorders forms the basis not only of accurate diagnosis but also of optimal management and care of individual dementia sufferers.

References

Cummings JL (1990) *Subcortical Dementia*. New York: Oxford University Press.

Dick JPR, Snowden JS, Northen B et al (1989) Slowly progressive apraxia. *Behav Neurol* **2:** 101–114.

Gibb WRG, Luthert PT, Marsden CD (1989) Corticobasal degeneration. *Brain* **112:** 1171–1192.

Gustafson L (1987) Frontal lobe degeneration of non-Alzheimer type. II. Clinical picture and differential diagnosis. *Arch Gerontol Geriatr* **6:** 209–223.

Harper P, Bates G, Jones L (2002) *Huntington's Disease.* Oxford: Oxford Medical Publications, 3rd edn.

Hutton M, Lendon CL, Rizzu P et al (1998) Association of missense and 5'-splice-site mutations in tau with the inherited dementia FTDP-17. *Nature* **393:** 702–705.

Lund and Manchester groups (1994) Consensus statement. Clinical and neuropathological criteria for fronto-temporal dementia. *J Neurol Neurosurg Psychiatry* **4:** 416–418.

Matthews WB (1985) Creutzfeldt–Jakob disease. In Frederiks JAM (ed) *Handbook of Clinical Neurology.* Amsterdam: Elsevier, pp 289–299.

McKeith IG, Galasko D, Kosaka K et al (1996) Consensus guidelines for the clinical and pathologic diagnosis of dementia with Lewy bodies (DLB): report of the consortium on DLB international workshop. *Neurology* **47:** 1113–1124.

McKhann G, Drachman D, Folstein M et al (1984) Clinical diagnosis of Alzheimer's disease: report of the NINCDS–ADRDA Work Group under the auspices of Department of Health and Human Services Task Force on Alzheimer's Disease. *Neurology* **34:** 939–944.

Neary D, Snowden JS, Gustafson L et al (1998) Frontotemporal lobar degeneration. A consensus on clinical diagnostic criteria. *Neurology* **51:** 1546–1554.

Riley DE, Lang AE, Lewis A et al (1990) Cortico-basal ganglionic degeneration. *Neurology* **40:** 1203–1212.

Snowden JS, Goulding PJ, Neary D (1989) Semantic dementia: a form of circumscribed atrophy. *Behav Neurol* **2:** 167–182.

Snowden JS, Neary D, Mann DMA (1996). *Fronto-temporal Lobar Degeneration: Fronto-temporal Dementia, Progressive Aphasia, Semantic Dementia.* New York: Churchill Livingstone.

Victor M, Adams RD, Collins GH (1971) *The Wernicke-Korsakoff Syndrome.* Oxford: Blackwell.

Will RG, Ironside JW, Zeidler M et al (1996) A new variant of Creutzfeldt–Jakob disease in the UK. *Lancet* **347:** 921–925.

Will RG, Zeidler M, Stewart GE et al (2000) Diagnosis of new variant Creutzfeldt–Jakob disease. *Ann Neurol* **47:** 575–582.

chapter 3

Assessment and referral

Robert Baldwin, Ruth Chaplin, Michelle Murray and Jackie Kindell

In this chapter we consider the assessments made by core members of the team, the psychiatrist, specialist nurse, occupational therapist, and speech and language therapist. This composition will vary from place to place and indeed since writing this, our own team has been enlarged by a social worker. The Manchester service, also called the 'Carisbrooke service', offers a multidisciplinary team approach to assessment. This should afford the younger person with a range of interventions that are relevant to their particular diagnosis and which should complement the diagnostic work. Roles in assessment, such as those of the psychologist and social worker, are discussed in Chapters 6 and 7. We begin with the psychiatrist, since in the Manchester service part of the psychiatrist's role is to screen referrals prior to assessment. Then, referral into the service is outlined, followed by the specific therapy assessments

Psychiatric assessment

The manifestations of dementia are threefold: *cognitive impairment*; *non-cognitive* symptoms (another term is 'behavioural and psychological symptoms in dementia' or BPSD); and *decrements in daily activity*

(Burns et al, 1999). The cognitive symptoms include memory difficulties, apraxia, geographical disorientation, aphasia, problems with writing and reading, along with difficulties in reasoning and making judgements. These are described in detail in Chapter 2.

Non-cognitive symptoms, or BPSD, will be discussed in most detail as they, at worst, lead to a breakdown of care or, at least, severe strain on families and caregivers. Those seeking further information about BPSD can access a well-produced modular series produced by the International Psychogeriatric Association (IPA) from its website (www.ipa-online.org).

There are five components to psychiatric evaluation: the history and mental state examination, risk assessment, physical examination, a range of physical investigations and identification of special factors. Each will be described in brief.

History and mental state

After recording the main symptoms, usually amplified by someone who knows the patient well, the history continues with duration and intensity of problems as well as any fluctuation in them. It is important to check for a previous history of mental illness and to find out what medication the person is taking and how much alcohol is regularly consumed.

Agitation is a term frequently used to describe a phenomenon with two elements: (1) psychological, the person feels restless inwardly, and (2) behavioural, the person displays observable restlessness, ranging from fidgeting to ceaseless pacing. It is not specific to dementia; for example, agitation is frequently reported in depressive disorder. The person's distress, whether or not he/she retains the ability to express it, is manifest.

Psychotic symptoms may be found in about 10–15% of people with dementia (Allen and Burns, 1995). Often, they can be linked to memory disturbance—for example, believing that a relative has concealed a purse or wallet which has been mislaid, but sometimes they appear to have no relationship to reality at all—for example, believing that neighbours are conspiring to oust the person from their home.

Hallucinations occur a little less often but are by no means uncommon. Realizing the oddity of the experience, patients may not reveal that they hallucinate unless asked directly. Hallucinations usually occur in the visual mode, for example, seeing groups of strangers in the home.

Misidentifications and duplication phenomena are not necessarily psychiatric symptoms, as they may arise directly from damage to cortical areas. However, they have much in common with psychotic symptoms and can be especially distressing, for example, believing that a partner has been replaced by a double, or that it is crucial to leave home because the 'real' home, resembling the current one, is in a different location.

Mood disorder covers depression, anxiety and mania. The latter is very uncommon in dementia although on rare occasions it may herald its onset. Anxiety is more common, especially in the early stages of a dementia. The person is fretful and apprehensive, may find it difficult to get to sleep, finds it difficult to relax and may experience muscle tension or autonomic anxiety (churning of the stomach, loose motions, etc). Depressive disorder affects about 15–20% of people with dementia (Allen and Burns, 1995) and depressive symptoms about 50% (Chapter 3). As depression is a condition that is often poorly detected, it is worth being aware of the main symptoms. In early dementia, it may not be difficult to diagnose as the person may be able to articulate the symptoms—low mood, lack of enjoyment, irritability, reduced appetite (often with attendant weight loss), poor concentration, feeling of anxiety, early morning wakening, reduced interest in sex, negative feelings about oneself and hopelessness, manifesting in some as suicidal thinking. In severe dementia, it may be considerably more difficult to diagnose. Often, the manifestations will be behavioural, such as restlessness, irritable behaviour, sleeplessness and food refusal.

Interpreted correctly, a screening questionnaire may aid in the diagnosis of depression. The Geriatric Depression Scale (GDS), as its name suggests, was validated on 'older' people, although the original research included people in their early 50s. It has the advantage of

45

having a yes/no format and has been found to be valid at least in those with mild-to-moderate dementia. The 15-item version is reproduced in Appendix 1. It has been translated into many languages and further information can be obtained from the GDS website (http://stanford.edu/~yesavage/ GDS.html). Depression is difficult to diagnose in patients with advanced dementia and it is advisable to seek advice from a colleague with psychiatric training.

Inappropriate behaviours, such as undressing, social or even sexual indiscretions and marked lack of judgement, are common in dementia that affects the frontal region of the brain. These are discussed in Chapter 2.

It is vital to find out if the person is still driving. Although there is some debate as to whether mild/early dementia is a bar to safe driving—with some suggestions that the person might be safe if he/she keeps to familiar routes and is accompanied – dementia is a notifiable condition, so in all cases the person or his/her representative should notify the relevant driving authority (in the UK, the DVLA). If the person refuses, then confidential reporting to the DVLA is advised. The DVLA can, if needed, arrange for a test of the person's driving abilities.

Risk assessment

A risk assessment should include whether the person is a risk to themselves, for example, because they lack insight into kitchen safety, or to others, because they insist on driving when they are unsafe. Whether dementia is a risk factor for suicide is not clear, although patients with early dementia should be regarded as being at increased risk. Risk assessment is covered in greater detail later in the chapter.

Physical examination

A general examination is carried out for three reasons. First, because people with dementia may have physical health problems that are not suspected, people with dementia may not exhibit usual health-seeking behaviour. An example is the uncomplaining patient with an ailment which would be very painful to most non-demented people. Second, medical problems that are known should be treated optimally, otherwise they merely add to the problem (an example is anaemia). Third, examination of the nervous system is an integral part of diagnosing what type of dementia is present. This is covered in Chapter 2.

Physical investigations

For similar reasons to those described above, a range of investigations should be performed in all younger people presenting with a dementia. This should include routinely a full blood count, erythrocyte sedimentation rate or equivalent, a biochemical profile, vitamin B_{12} and folate estimates, and thyroid function tests. In addition, other tests, such as a chest X-ray and electrocardiogram may be requested, depending on clinical findings. Each person presenting with dementia should receive a brain scan which might be a computed tomography (CT) or, increasingly, a magnetic resonance imaging (MRI) scan. Nowadays, these are not arduous tests although they do require a certain amount of cooperation so that someone who knows the person should be on hand. SPECT (single-photon emission CT) scanning has been mentioned in Chapter 2. This is available in departments of nuclear medicine in many larger hospitals. It requires an injection of radioactive contrast dye. It measures blood perfusion and can be very helpful in differentiating types of dementia.

Special factors

Some dementias affecting younger people, for example, Huntington's disease, some forms of early onset Alzheimer's disease and some cases of frontal lobe dementia, have a genetic basis. It is vital to be able to refer to clinical geneticists who can discuss the implication of these disorders with family members. In Manchester, the Clinical Genetics department is located in a nearby hospital and has developed considerable expertise with younger onset dementias.

Clearly, the assessment of a younger person with dementia requires specialist knowledge. When planning services for this age group it is very important to identify within the locality who has such skills. Often, it will be the neurological services but increasingly in the UK, old age psychiatrists also have had the necessary training. Another route into an assessment is the local memory clinic, which may offer a comprehensive assessment (Chapter 12).

Referral into the service

Once a person has received a diagnosis of dementia (frequently a difficult and prolonged process), the individual and his/her family are often left not knowing what services, if any, are available. We have discussed (Chapter 1) why specialist provision for the younger person is helpful. He/she may be, or have recently been, in work and now has considerable frustration at being inactive; may have young dependent children and need child care provision; and may have carers who need to work, especially as there are often financial commitments such as mortgage payments.

Referral criteria
We have laid down eligibility criteria for the Carisbrooke service:

■ a person between the ages of 18 and 64 years,
■ with a confirmed diagnosis of dementia,
■ living within the City of Manchester.

We believe that these conditions are fair, transparent and not overly restrictive. For example, many people referred to us, especially in the early years, had not received adequate investigations. We think that having strict criteria about a confirmed diagnosis contributes to raising standards rather than merely being awkward. Having said that, anyone can make a referral to the service using a single telephone number. Our aim is to assist and fully inform the younger person with dementia about any relevant information that is beneficial to them. It can also assist people with access to relevant investigations and assessments for diagnosis. Some specialist services for younger people in the UK only accept referrals for conditions that are progressive. This may lead to other conditions, such as Korsakoff syndrome, being excluded. It was decided by the Carisbrooke service that these people would not be excluded but that acceptance would be based on need (i.e. person-based rather than diagnosis-oriented). In an area such as inner-city Manchester there are many people who have cognitive impairment due to alcohol. The younger persons' dementia service has become a lifeline for many of them. However, we can accept that where services are pressed to ration what they provide, then sometimes the diagnosis can be brought into the equation. For example, the Carisbrooke service is reluctant to take patients with learning disability because the Learning Disability Service has greater skills in the general management of such individuals even though it has less direct experience of dementia.

All new referrals are discussed at weekly team meetings. A decision is taken on whether to accept the referral, and whether to offer a service or provide advice. Sometimes, the response is to seek further information. The psychiatrist in the team will often write asking for clarification about diagnosis or suggesting a referral to the Cerebral Function Unit or the Memory Clinic to make a diagnosis. Otherwise, a named member of the team will make the initial contact with the person referred and the referrer.

Initial service assessment

We recommend using a standardized, structured tool for the first assessment. The Carisbrooke service uses a bespoke assessment tool—the Manchester Care Assessment Schedule (MANCAS; Firth, 1998). This provides an assessment of health and social needs and is used by all mental health staff in Manchester. It has the advantage that an assessment conducted by a mental health professional accessing the service need not be repeated. MANCAS includes an assessment of risk both to self and others and of environmental risk. The aim is to complete this over the first two meetings with the user and their carer. However, when the user lives alone this is not always possible. From the information gathered, the person's strengths and his/her needs should be established leading to allocation of a member of the team who will act as 'key worker'. Other services may use different terms—

in Manchester, the latter refers to someone who will ensure that care is coordinated. It does not mean that the key worker is responsible for purchasing packages of care, although this could be possible if the organizational arrangements were in place, such as pooling of budgets with social services.

The Care Programme Approach (CPA): CPA reviews and service reviews

The CPA was introduced in 1993 with the aim of focusing the provision of care and support received on the needs of the person receiving them (NHSE/SSI, 1999). In England, the CPA applies to all people accepted by specialist services and its main requirements are:

- An assessment of the service user's health and social care needs, including an assessment of any risks posed by them or to them.
- A multidisciplinary care plan stating how the assessed care needs are going to be met.
- Appointment of a key worker to oversee the implementation of the care plan and to involve the appropriate services.
- Regular reviews to ensure the continuing appropriateness of the care plan.
- The involvement of the service user in the process.

In the Manchester Younger Persons Dementia Service, about half the users accepted have CPA key workers based in another service (e.g. general psychiatry), and in the other half the key worker is a member of the specialist team. The decision about who takes on this role depends on user preference, complexity of the case and how many other agencies are involved. As we do not attempt to replicate mainstream services, complex cases may be better served by having care coordinated from within such a mainstream service. We often host CPA reviews at Carisbrooke and attend CPA reviews of our other users that are held elsewhere.

> **Case Study**
>
> Elizabeth was referred to the service in March 2000 by her husband. She was then 59 years old and had a diagnosis of Alzheimer's disease. Her husband was in full-time employment and had some support from their daughters and friends. Elizabeth had been given her diagnosis by the Manchester Memory Clinic (see Chapter 12) in 1998 and prescribed an antidepressant and a cholinesterase inhibitor (Chapter 4). Ongoing monitoring was by a nurse and consultant psychogeriatrician based in her locality, the latter acting as key worker. The Carisbrooke specialist nurse carried out the MANCAS assessment and the occupational therapist also performed appropriate assessments both at home and at the day care centre in Carisbrooke. From this service, care plans were formulated that centred on the preservation of Elizabeth's social skills and opportunities to continue creative and productive activities. Elizabeth was offered day care at Carisbrooke one day a week and an afternoon of outreach care from one of our support workers.
>
> CPA reviews were hosted by Carisbrooke and members of the Manchester Memory Clinic attended along with Elizabeth and her family. Care plans were reviewed and the need to involve other agencies was identified. In 2001, a referral was made to the Adult Placement Service (a mainstream service offering individual day care, respite or long-term care either in the worker's home or the client's home), for additional home support for Elizabeth and an extra day of day care was offered. Regular reviews continue to evaluate and update CPA care plans with the other agencies involved and with Elizabeth and her family.

Nursing assessment

After the initial assessment using MANCAS, there is usually a clearer understanding of which disciplines need to complete further assessments. McLennan (1999) suggests that, in particular, the younger person with dementia will often experience:

- symptoms of anxiety and depression,
- personality change with blunting of emotional perception and responsiveness,
- development, at times, of paranoid ideas.

A local study (Ferran et al, 1996) identified that almost half of a large sample of younger people with dementia had experienced symptoms of depression and almost one-third had symptoms of challenging behaviour. McLennan (1999) also suggests that the person with dementia can feel that something is wrong even though he/she cannot understand what it is. Usually, the person closest first notices the changes so that it is vital to speak to him/her. In the Manchester service we find that the younger person with dementia often feels more relieved when difficulties are discussed openly and honestly. This leads to a major role for the nurse in working with family members to help them come to terms with the effects of the illness and changes in family roles (see also Chapter 11). Discussions will usually include the younger person with dementia.

Following a diagnosis of dementia, families are often left feeling stunned and bewildered. Many feel that they need more information concerning the condition. Others often find that questions arise in the days or weeks following diagnosis of dementia. Individuals need to build trusting relationships with a nurse so that a mutual therapeutic relationship can be developed. People often need to discuss issues such as vulnerability, competence, sexuality and intimacy. Sometimes families can become 'stuck' or have difficulty resolving issues; on these occasions we would refer people to the Family Therapy Team (Chapter 11).

Risk assessment

The risk assessment is a requirement for every individual for whom a referral is accepted. The areas that are assessed in the local service include:

1 Risk factors

2 History

3 Ideation

4 Plans

5 Intent

6 Protective factors

7 Summary:

  (a) what is the patient at risk of?

  (b) what is the severity of the risk?

  (c) what is the timescale of that risk (i.e. immediate, short term, long term)?

Based on the findings of the risk assessment, the individual practitioner will exercise clinical judgement to decide the most appropriate immediate course of action. A risk-management strategy should be formulated on the basis of risk factors versus protective factors as identified above. Many of the referrals we have received have been from medical wards at one of the three local general hospitals. Although Carisbrooke does not offer a diagnostic service, other health service professionals often have little or no experience in the symptomatology or service needs of the younger person with dementia. Thus, a consultation service based on assessment and/or advice is offered to patients deemed to be 'bed blocking'.

Occupational therapy assessment

The framework used for assessment and intervention is the Canadian Model of Occupational Performance (CAOT, 1997). In this model, people are seen as active and occupational by nature and their activities are determined by their perceived roles and responsibilities and the influence of the culture and society in which they live. A state of well-being will be maintained by the person achieving a balance of activities in the areas of self-care (activities to maintain the individual such as cooking, eating, washing and dressing), productivity (activities to maintain the environment or acquire sustenance such as preparing food for others, unpaid or paid work) and leisure (activities to fulfil a person's own creative or aesthetic needs such as hobbies and socializing). Therefore, occupational therapy assessment will explore a person's performance in these areas, discuss what his/her priorities and motivations are, and from this information plan relevant interventions.

Assessment of activities of daily living

Following the initial interview in which the necessary background information will be gathered from the person and their carer, where relevant, the occupational therapist will proceed to carry out a functional assessment. This is best performed in the person's home environment as this is the one they are most familiar with. The aim of this assessment with younger people who have dementia is to gather information to provide a basis on which to identify the person's strengths and needs.

Functional assessment should be carried out over two visits if possible, as the occupational performance of a person with dementia may vary from day to day. As with all persons who have dementia, it is important to see the person performing activities on his/her own without the caregiver, as this is the only way to gain a clear picture of what his/her skills are. Only relevant activities should be assessed. For example, if the person has never cooked a meal and has no need to cook a meal then assessing the person performing this unfamiliar task is not useful and may only serve to distress them. Younger people with dementia often have insight into the difficulties that they are experiencing in daily living tasks but do not like to discuss these as they may feel embarrassed or afraid. It is very important that the therapist explain that the aim of the assessment is to look at ways of adapting tasks to enable continued independence and/or to adapt the environment.

Leisure activities profile

This explores the structure of the client's day and week, their past and present interests and what they perceive as preventing them from carrying out activities. It is very useful in building up a good rapport with clients as they are talking about the things that are meaningful in their life. By looking at the structure of their day and dividing activities into self-care, productivity and leisure, the therapist can see where intervention to redress the balance of activity are needed. Information from carergivers and/or friends and other professionals is very important in these areas of assessment, and the occupational therapist will also take into account the needs of the carergiver when carrying out assessment and planning interventions.

Standardized assessments of cognitive functioning

Standardized assessments are used to monitor levels of deterioration and also to identify and minimize the risk to patients and clients. Often, the assessment tools that are available can be inadequate due to the nature of symptoms presented. For example, a person with visuospatial impairment will be unable to perform the Pentagon test on the Mini-Mental State Examination (MMSE; Folstein et al, 1973). However, other areas of the MMSE may highlight little or no difficulty with other categories such as calculation and recall.

Standardized tools may also be useful in pinpointing areas of need and precise areas of impairment and may complement the less formal approach of the other occupational therapy assessments. They include AMPS (Assessment of Motor and Process Skills), the Bristol Activities of Daily Living (ADL) scale, SOTOF (Structured Observational Test of Function) and LACLS (Large Allen Cognitive Level Screen; Allen, 1996). The latter is based on Piaget's model of cognitive development and is useful in planning appropriate activities for those with various levels of functional ability.

Speech and language therapy assessment

Communication disorders may initially present with very mild problems particularly in verbal expression and writing. However, difficulties increase in these areas together with problems of comprehension and reading as the dementia progresses. In the later stages communication may be significantly impaired. It is important to remember that different types of dementia present with different patterns of communication impairment (Chapter 2). A comprehensive range of assessments is therefore required to analyse these problems, and these are available within most dysphasia resources. However, it is also vital to assess the contribution that other cognitive areas make to communication breakdown. Most importantly, assessment of immediate, recent and long-term memory should be carried out. Assessment may be carried out on an individual or group basis. A vital component of this will be analysis of functional communication, particularly with relatives and caregivers, and in this context conversational analysis techniques will be useful.

Assessment of swallowing may be through formal dysphagia assessment; however, many individuals may be unable to cooperate with this as such problems tend to present in the later stages of dementia. Therefore, observation of the person and the environment at mealtimes may be more appropriate (Kindell, 2002).

References

Allen CK (1996) *Large Allen Cognitive Level Screen Test Manual.* Colchester, CT, USA: S & S Worldwide.

Allen NHP, Burns A (1995) The non-cognitive features of dementia. *Rev Clin Gerontology* **5:** 57–75.

Burns A, Russell E, Page S (1999) New drugs for Alzheimer's Disease. *Br J Psychiatry* **174:** 476–479.

CAOT (Canadian Association of Occupational Therapists) (1997) *Enabling Occupation: an Occupational Therapy Perspective.* Ottawa: CAOT Publications, p 32.

Ferran J, Wilson K, Doran M (1996) The early onset dementia: a study of clinical characteristics and service use. *Int J Geriatr Psychiatry* **11:** 863–869.

Firth MT (1998) *The Manchester Care Assessment Schedule*. Manchester Psychiatric Social Work Educational Centre. University of Manchester.

Folstein MF, Folstein SE, McHugh PR (1975) 'Mini-Mental State': a practical method for grading the cognitive state of patients for the clinician. *J Psychiatr Res* **12:** 189–198.

Kindell J (2002) *Feeding and Swallowing Disorders in Dementia*. Bicester, UK: Speechmark Publishing.

McLennan J (1999) In Cox S, Keady J (eds) *Younger People with Dementia: Planning, Practice and Development*. London/Philadelphia: Jessica Kingsley, p 17.

NHSE/SSI (National Health Service Executive/Social Services Inspectorate) (1999) *Effective Care Co-ordination in Mental Health*. London: NHSE Publications.

Neary D (1999) Classification of the dementias. *Rev Clin Gerontology* **9:** 55–64.

chapter 4

Treatments for dementia

Robert Baldwin and Sean Page

Non-pharmacological management

The disparate terms covering problem behaviours and phenomena in dementia include 'non-cognitive symptoms' and 'behavioural and psychological symptoms of dementia' (BPSD). For a detailed guide to the non-pharmacological treatment of BPSD, the reader should consult the International Psychogeriatric Association (IPA) website (www.ipa-online.org/). The BPSD teaching modules can be downloaded, including one devoted to this topic. In addition, although written largely for carergivers of older people with dementia, the book by Mace and Rabins (1991) remains a classic resource for anyone struggling with the demands of caregiving.

Here, the principles of non-pharmacological management will be described. More detail and illustrations are found in Emma Shlosberg's Chapter 6. Non-pharmacological interventions are usually first-line in dealing with milder behavioural and psychological symptoms of dementia (Teri et al, 1992), although there is limited research supporting the use of many interventions. For moderate to severe BPSD, medication is often indicated although it should not automatically be prescribed. This is discussed later.

Symptoms that are most responsive to non-pharmacological interventions include:

- mild depression/apathy,
- wandering/pacing,
- repetitive questioning/mannerisms.

Environmental factors are frequent causes and contributors to BPSD. The ideal environment for a patient with dementia is one that is non-stressful, constant and familiar. Sudden changes to the environment should be avoided, or where inevitable, likely behavioural sequelae should be recognized (e.g. wandering away from a new environment to look for the old familiar one).

A general approach to behavioural interventions includes:
- Identifying the target BPSD (e.g. wandering).
- Gathering information about it.
- Identifying the triggers or consequential events of a specific symptom.
- Setting realistic goals and making plans.
- Encouraging caregivers to reward themselves and others for achieving goals.
- Continually evaluating and modifying plans.

Recreational, music and bright-light therapies are interventions that have been shown to reduce anxiety and agitation in other populations, and which are sometimes used with dementia patients. Psychological interventions including psychotherapy (individual, group and family) may be useful, particularly in the early stages of dementia. For further information see Chapters 6 and 11.

Pharmacological treatment for dementia

Such is the devastating personal impact of dementia that any mention of treatment invariably raises hopes and produces expectations that are often unrealistic. If one considers the concept of cure as being the only truly effective treatment then in the field of dementia, it remains as elusive as ever. If, however, one takes a more pragmatic view then it may be suggested that, in part, it has always been possible to treat the symptoms of dementia. Antidepressants may be used to treat symptoms of depression in people with dementia whilst the neuroleptics (antipsychotics, major tranquillizers) are helpful in reducing aggression, agitation or delusions, when first-line non-pharmacological strategies, such as those already discussed, fail. We have devoted quite a lot of space to cholinesterase inhibitors. This is not to overstate their place in helping younger people with dementia but to emphasize the importance of having sound up-to-date knowledge, for they frequently come up in discussion with both the person with dementia and their caregivers.

The cholinesterase inhibitors

At the present time, attention is focused upon the recently emerging class of drugs known as the cholinesterase inhibitors (ChEIs). These drugs represent an important shift in our thinking about Alzheimer's disease and offer, for the first time, the potential to be therapeutically active against the symptoms of dementia and their rate of progression. However, before considering the ChEIs it is important to set them in their scientific context and to consider the rationale for treatment.

Cholinergic functioning

A growing body of empirical evidence is highlighting the neurochemical deficits of Alzheimer's disease and there is a significant focus upon the cholinergic system and its principal neurotransmitter acetylcholine (ACh). ACh is highly influential in processes of memory and learning and after having crossed the synapse it is hydrolysed, broken down, by the acetylcholinesterase enzyme. The cholinergic hypothesis (Bartus et al, 1982) suggests that a selective loss of cholinergic neurons brings about reduced levels of ACh in Alzheimer's disease, progressively disabling cognitive functioning.

More recently, attention has focused upon the involvement of a second enzyme, butanoylcholinesterase, which also exerts a hydrolysing effect on ACh (Massoulie, 2000) and the inhibition of which not only raises levels of available ACh but also produces fewer side-effects, at least in animal studies. It is possible that inhibiting butanoylcholinesterase could have therapeutic effects in severe Alzheimer's disease where this enzyme is found in higher quantities than acetylcholinesterase.

Developing a greater understanding of the underlying pathophysiology has led to the concept of preserving cognition, in mild-to-moderate Alzheimer's disease, by seeking ways to maintain existing levels of ACh. Targeting the acetylcholinesterase enzyme and inhibiting its action has become the preferred option and from this the first generation antidementia drugs, the ChEIs, have been introduced.

Each of the three ChEIs currently licensed and available for clinical use, and the many others that have been or are currently being developed, act in a slightly different way from each other. Sim (1999) has described these differences. Some have an irreversible action in that they inactivate the enzyme completely until it is slowly replaced, over a number of weeks, by a newly synthesized enzyme. Others are reversible, meaning that they achieve only very weak ionic bonds with acetylcholinesterase and these bonds are quickly broken. As a consequence, it is only possible to achieve inhibition of action for a very short period of time. Finally, some ChEIs are pseudo-reversible meaning that once the drug binds with the enzyme it is rapidly hydrolysed whilst remaining attached and consequently inactivating the enzyme. This is an elegant mechanism which results in the drug being quickly destroyed at the site of action whilst inhibiting the enzyme for a sufficiently long period.

Donepezil (Aricept)

The first of the ChEIs to be licensed for the treatment of mild-to-moderate Alzheimer's disease, donepezil, is available in a once-daily dose of 5 mg or 10 mg. It is a reversible inhibitor that circumvents the short duration of inhibition by virtue of a long plasma half-life of some 70 hours. Donepezil is selective of acetylcholinesterase, bringing about upwards of 90% inhibition at its maximum dose of

10 mg per day (Nordberg and Svensson, 1998) although it has a much more limited effect upon butanoylcholinesterase.

Clinical trials have reported benefits in cognitive functioning in comparison with placebo (Rogers et al, 1998). In a later trial (Doody et al, 2001) it was found that treatment of up to 144 weeks conferred benefit. All reported clinical trials have shown the treatment group to have significant improvements in cognitive functioning in comparison to the placebo group.

Donepezil may cause side-effects although most are clinically mild and transient in nature. Those commonly reported are nausea, vomiting, loose stools, muscle cramping, insomnia, fatigue and dizziness. Side-effects most commonly occur within a two-week period when treatment is first initiated or after the dose has been increased. Cost of treatment ranges from £890 to £1250 per patient per annum (UK costs in 2001).

Rivastigmine (Exelon)

Rivastigmine is described as a centrally selective inhibitor of acetylcholinesterase; it is believed to be highly selective for brain areas such as the cortex and hippocampus, where much cholinergic activity occurs. It has also been shown to have a dual inhibitory function with an additional impact upon butanoylcholinesterase (Nordberg and Svensson, 1998). Because of its pseudo-irreversible effect it has a relatively short half-life of one hour (Sim, 1999).

Depending on one's point of view, the dosing regime is either more complex or more flexible than for donepezil. If taken as a single dose, rivastigmine would only inhibit cholinesterase activity for up to 10 hours, so that it is recommended to be taken twice a day. There are four doses available: 1.5 mg bd, 3 mg bd, 4.5 mg bd and 6 mg bd. Whilst this does offer greater dosing flexibility to suit individual patient needs it may reduce compliance. Cost of treatment, regardless of dose, is £821 per individual patient per annum (UK costs in 2001).

Clinical trial data has shown that rivastigmine has a consistently significant benefit over placebo in terms of cognition and activities of daily living. This effect is greatest for higher doses, 6–12 mg per day.

Most trial data has been pooled from the original research programme and analyses are based on trials of several thousands. Much smaller pilot studies have also reported positive effects in terms of the behavioural and psychiatric symptoms of dementia.

McKeith et al (2000) have reported a trial of rivastigmine in 120 patients with Lewy body dementia and found significant benefit in respect of attention and psychotic symptoms. Early data has suggested benefit in nursing home residents with behavioural disturbance caused by severe dementia. This therapeutic effect in severe dementia may be related to the inhibition of butanoylcholinesterase.

The side-effect profile of rivastigmine is similar to the other ChEIs despite its claim to be selective to the central nervous system. The higher doses, whilst offering greater potential for benefit, also offer the greater risk of side-effects, of which the most common are nausea, vomiting, loose stools, weight loss, anorexia, insomnia, fatigue and dizziness.

Galantamine (Reminyl)

Galantamine, a reversible inhibitor predominantly of acetyl-cholinesterase, exerts only limited effect on butanoylcholinesterase, but has a dual effect of modulating nicotinic cholinergic receptors. The other ChEIs have no effect upon nicotinic receptors. This modulating effect may permit a greater amount of ACh to be released at the synapse and may therefore potentially offer a different profile of clinical activity or patient response.

The dosing regime again is of twice-daily administration and again there are a number of doses available for titration. Galantamine is available as 4 mg bd, 8 mg bd or 12 mg bd. The cost of treatment is from £785 to £1204 per patient per annum (UK costs in 2001).

Upwards of 2000 patients have participated in clinical trials involving galantamine. The results again are suggestive of statistically significant improvements, over placebo, in respect of cognition and activities of daily living. The side-effect profile is similar to the other ChEIs and is again greater at higher doses.

Clinical application of cholinesterase inhibitors

The ChEIs are a welcome addition to the management package of Alzheimer's disease offering the potential for some people to experience a period of stability. This stability allows other non-pharmacological therapeutic activities targeted at caregiver support and maximizing patient potential to be introduced. The use of the ChEIs is, however, subject to national guidelines which make their introduction to clinical practice potentially complicated and resource-heavy.

In England, the National Institute for Clinical Excellence (NICE) has produced guidance on the use of the ChEIs (NICE, 2001). At the present time these guidelines reflect the product licences, and only cover mild-to-moderate Alzheimer's disease. They therefore begin by stating that before treatment with a ChEI may be initiated, a diagnosis of Alzheimer's disease must be made following specialist assessment and investigation and based upon standardized diagnostic criteria.

Following this, treatment under a specialist may then be initiated, with the specialist team assuming responsibility for subsequent monitoring, although a shared care protocol for prescribing may be developed with primary care practitioners. The role of the specialist is to monitor patients' response to treatment, to advise on changes to the dosing regime, and to advise about when to discontinue the medication. The usual reasons for stopping treatment are poor compliance, poor tolerance, poor efficacy or a change in health status of the person with dementia.

Treatment may be continued whilst the patient is objectively seen to derive benefit from doing so. One of the controversial issues about treatment has been when and how to assess whether it is working. Early advice (Standing Medical Advisory Committee, 1998) recommended review after three months with a decision made at that point about efficacy. NICE has perhaps accepted that this is too early and recommends a first review once the patient has been on an effective dose for two to four months. Because of the longer titration regimes required for the twice-daily ChEIs this amounts to a recommendation for formal review and decision-making at approximately six months after initiating treatment.

It is suggested (Adams and Page, 2000) that treatment response be assessed across four domains, namely:

1 cognitive functioning,
2 participation in activities of daily living,
3 the frequency and severity of psychopathology,
4 a global impression of change.

The occurrence of side-effects in some people on treatment may be a factor that results in poor compliance. NICE suggests that a mechanism to ensure compliance should be in place before treatment is initiated. Probably, the most appropriate compliance mechanism is the permanent presence of a cohabitee, usually spouse, partner or child, who is prepared to accept responsibility for supervising treatment day to day. This becomes more problematic when patients live alone, although this is less likely with younger people with dementia. Where it does occur, an option is to prescribe donepezil and to provide a regular daily medication prompt via the Social Services.

The service response to these guidelines has been the introduction of the dementia treatment clinic model (Chapter 12), which has responsibility for managing the use of the ChEI within specific domains, to:

■ assess suitability for treatment,
■ initiate prescription of a ChEI,
■ monitor individual patient response,
■ stop treatment when indicated.

In Manchester, there has been a treatment clinic since 1997 following the licensing of donepezil. Experience has been gained with all three of the licensed drugs. Younger people are included and are referred by the Younger Persons Dementia Service. Global benefit is assessed using a Clinical Global Impression of Change Scale. With this scale, collated evidence of efficacy is weighed alongside the clinical judgement of the patient and a degree of benefit assigned as an improvement (mild, moderate or marked); no change from baseline; or

Table 4.1 Degree of benefit from a ChEI over a 12-month period (n = 85)

	% showing benefit from treatment with ChEI	% showing no benefit from treatment with ChEI
3 months	88.2	11.8
6 months	76.7	22.3
12 months	68.3	31.7

deterioration (mild, moderate or marked). This naturalistic data based on local experience is presented in Table 4.1 and shows that treatment with a ChEI is of benefit to the majority of patients, including those with a younger age of onset of Alzheimer's disease.

Future directions in treatment with antidementia agents

Although the ChEIs represent the first generation of drug treatments for Alzheimer's disease the search for the next generations continues. The following are all possible future directions:

- Extending the use of the ChEIs.
- Using agents with protective or preventive properties.
- Introducing novel therapeutic agents.

For example, at the time of writing (2003), memantine, for use in severe dementia, has been licensed in the UK. It acts by blocking the excess release of the neurotransmitter glutamate. It may be used when existing ChEIs cannot be tolerated or in combination with a ChEI, although more data are needed on the effectiveness of combining treatments. Efficacy studies are beginning to be reported, including in vascular dementia (Wilcock, 2000).

Extended product licences

At the time of writing, the ChEIs are only licensed for the treatment of mild-to-moderate Alzheimer's disease. Research data, as yet unpublished, is alluding to the possibility of extended licences for treatment of the dementias associated with cerebrovascular disease and for severe dementia. Clinical trials continue to explore the therapeutic potential in mild cognitive impairment and Lewy body dementia, amongst others. Considering the mode of action of the ChEIs it is quite likely that product licences for all three agents may be extended over the course of the next few years.

Protective or preventative agents

Early research trials, with some methodological flaws, have suggested that agents such as vitamin E may delay the onset of Alzheimer's disease by almost a year (Sano et al, 1997).

Epidemiological studies of anti-inflammatory agents, such as indomethacin, have reported that they may delay the onset of dementia or slow its progression. McGeer et al (1996) reviewed 17 such studies and found a positive effect, in that the risk of developing Alzheimer's disease could be reduced by about 50%.

Oestrogens have been considered in a number of limited studies. Some early evidence suggests that replacement therapy may act to delay the onset and severity of dementia (Jones, 2000). However, progress in all these areas is at an early stage and carers and those with dementia should not be misled by over-optimistic reports.

Novel therapeutic agents

Scientific attention in recent years has moved away from focusing exclusively on the cholinergic deficit of Alzheimer's disease to explore alternative treatment possibilities. In particular, the potential for an immunosuppressant vaccine has been tentatively reported, but at the time of writing cases of acute encephalopathy have led to trials being halted.

Antipsychotic agents

There are two broad categories of antipsychotic (neuroleptic) medications available for use in dementia patients:

1 Conventional neuroleptics are primarily dopamine D_2-blockers and are associated with the development of extrapyramidal side-effects (EPS). Examples include haloperidol and promazine. Another agent that was widely and perhaps indiscriminately used, thioridazine, was recently restricted for use because of concerns about sudden cardiac death.

2 The second category is newer and is often referred to as novel or atypical, as this class of agent is not usually associated with EPS. These agents have weak D_2-blocking potential or, if they have D_2-antagonist properties, these are balanced by serotonergic antagonist action. Clozapine was the first and prototypical novel antipsychotic but there are now a number of agents available, including risperidone, olanzapine and quetiapine.

These newer so-called atypical antipsychotic agents (risperidone, olanzapine, quetiapine) are much safer and are now agents of first choice for psychosis associated with Alzheimer's disease and other dementias. However, they do not have product licences for the treatment of non-specific agitation in dementia. In our experience, however, in carefully selected patients their use can be very beneficial to those afflicted with severe agitation that is non-responsive to non-pharmacological approaches, although it is preferable that this be done in association with a specialist and regular review of the medication. Based on the evidence (Devanand et al, 1989), the symptoms that appear to be most responsive to neuroleptic medications are:

- physical aggression and violent behaviours,
- psychosis (hallucinations, delusions),
- hostility.

Of the randomized, placebo-controlled trials of conventional neu-roleptics in dementia patients, most had small numbers of patients and were of short duration. Consistent findings in these studies (Devanand, 1995) were:

- frequent occurrence of side-effects,
- a large placebo effect,
- variable efficacy.

To date, two large multicentre trials with risperidone in BPSD have been conducted. Risperidone at a dose of 1 mg/day has been found to be superior to placebo in the treatment of BPSD, particularly for aggressive behaviours in dementia patients, but also for psychotic symptoms. Risperidone at this dose is well tolerated and has an EPS profile similar to placebo (Brecher, 1997; De Deyn, 1997). Reports on the tolerability to novel antipsychotics such as risperidone in patients with dementia with Lewy bodies have been both positive and negat-ive (McKeith et al, 1995). Table 4.2 reproduces the recommendations of the International Psychogeriatric Association (IPA) on the treatment of BPSD (as on the IPA website: www.ipa-online.org/).

Table 4.2 Clinical recommendations for the doses of conventional neuroleptics and newer antipsychotics in the treatment of BPSD

Drug	Start (mg)	Dose range (mg)	Schedule
Haloperidol	0.5	0.5–2	Once or twice daily
Thiothixene	1	1–10	Once daily
Risperidone	0.5	0.5–2	Once daily
*Clozapine**	6.25	10–100	Once or twice daily
Olanzapine	5	5–10	Once daily

*May require haematological monitoring.

Benzodiazepines

BPSDs that respond best to benzodiazepines include:

■ Anxiety
■ Tension
■ Irritability
■ Insomnia

Short-acting benzodiazepines, such as oxazepam or lorazepam, that do not accumulate are to be preferred. Low doses (e.g. lorazepam 0.5–2.0 mg/day) should be used for a limited-time period. Lorazepam may be especially useful as a premedication for episodic disturbance or where agitation or distress can be anticipated (e.g. minor surgical procedure or dental visit).

Antidepressants

There is a high rate of placebo response in studies of antidepressants given to patients with dementia. With this in mind, for those with mild depressive symptoms it is best to offer support to the patient and caregiver and review the situation over the following 4 weeks (the time within which most placebo responders have occurred in therapeutic trials).

If an antidepressant is to be prescribed, selective serotonin reuptake inhibitors (SSRIs) or secondary amine tricyclic antidepressants should be used. Doses should start low and be increased gradually as tolerated. A dosing schedule for selected antidepressants is shown in Table 4.3. Patients should be treated for a limited time period (usually 6 months) and do not necessarily need to be maintained on antidepressants indefinitely, as many of the depressions remit within a 12-month period.

It is recommended that antidepressants be given with supportive psychotherapy to the patient along with focused caregiver support. There is some evidence that SSRIs are effective in reducing symptoms

71

Table 4.3 Dosing schedule for selected antidepressants in patients with dementia

Drug	Initial dose (mg/day)	Target dose (mg/day)
Paroxetine	10	20–30
Fluoxetine	10	20–30
Sertraline	25	50–100
Nortriptyline	10	20–60
Moclobemide	150	150–600
Mirtazepine	15	15–45

in dementia, such as agitation and food refusal, which may have their basis in affective disorder, although there are no randomized controlled clinical trials. In some, but not all studies, improvement in cognition has been observed after depression in dementia has been treated.

Conclusion

The dementia syndrome has always been partially treatable with symptomatic therapies. The emergence of the ChEIs has introduced the potential to treat the cognitive symptoms of dementia whilst also having some impact on behavioural symptoms and activities of daily living. Other approaches using antipsychotic (neuroleptic) medication and antidepressants have a limited but useful place in the pharmacological management of dementia. ChEIs represent a first generation of newer treatment and their use remains subject to national guidance and specialist administration. Despite this they highlight that conditions, such as Alzheimer's disease, are potentially treatable. They may well have a positive impact upon the negative attitudes and nihilism that have permeated dementia care for far too long.

References

Adams T, Page SC (2000) New pharmacological treatments for Alzheimer's disease: implications for dementia care nursing. *J Adv Nurs* **31:** 1183–1188.

Bartus RT, Dean RL, Beer B et al (1982) The cholinergic hypothesis of geriatric memory dysfunction. *Science* **217:** 408–417.

Brecher M (1997) Risperidone in the treatment of psychosis and aggressive behaviour in patients with dementia. Paper presented at the Congress of the International Psychogeriatric Association (IPA), Jerusalem, Israel, 17–22 August.

Burns A, Russell E, Page S (1999) New drugs for Alzheimer's disease. *Br J Psychiatry* **174:** 476–479.

De Deyn P. (1997) Risperidone in the treatment of behavioural disturbances in dementia. Paper presented at the Congress of the International Psychogeriatric Association (IPA), Jerusalem, Israel, 17–22 August.

Devanand DP (1995) Role of neuroleptics in treatment of behavioral complications. In Lawlor BA (ed) *Behavioral Complications in Alzheimer's Disease*. Washington, DC: APA Press.

Devanand D, Sackheim HA, Brown R et al (1989) A pilot study of haloperidol treatment of psychosis and behavioral disturbance in Alzheimer's disease. *Arch Neurol* **46:** 854–857.

Doody RS, Geldmacher DS, Gordon B et al (2001) Open-label, multicenter, phase 3 extension study of the safety and efficacy of Donepezil in patients with Alzheimer's disease. *Arch Neurol* **58:** 427-433.

Jones R (2000) *Drug Treatment in Dementia*. Oxford, UK: Blackwell Science.

Mace NL, Rabins RV (1991) *The 36-hour day: A Family Guide to Caring for Persons with Alzheimer's Disease, Related Dementing Illnesses, and Memory Loss in Later Life*. Baltimore: Johns Hopkins University Press.

Massoulie J (2000) Molecular forms and anchoring of acetylcholinesterase. In Giacobini E (ed) *Cholinesterases and Cholinesterase Inhibitors*. London: Martin Dunitz.

McGeer PL, Schulzer M, McGeer EG (1996) Arthritis and anti-inflammatory agents as possible protective factors for Alzheimer's disease: a review of 17 epidemiological studies. *Neurology* **47:** 425–432.

McKeith IG, Ballard CG, Harrison RW (1995) Neuroleptic sensitivity to risperidone in Lewy body dementia. *Lancet* **346:** 699.

McKeith IG, Del Ser T, Spano PF et al (2000) Efficacy of rivastigmine in dementia with Lewy bodies: a randomised double-blind, placebo-controlled international study. *Lancet* **356:** 2031–2036.

NICE (National Institute for Clinical Excellence) (2001) *Technology Appraisal Guidance Number 19: Guidance on the use of donepezil, rivastigmine and galantamine for the treatment of Alzheimer's disease*. London: NICE.

Nordberg A, Svensson AL (1998) Cholinesterase inhibitors in the treatment of Alzheimer's disease: a comparison of tolerability and pharmacology. *Drug Safety* **19:** 465–480.

Rogers SL, Farlow MR, Doody RS (1998) A 24 week, double-blind, placebo controlled trial of donepezil in patients with Alzheimer's disease. *Neurology* **50:** 136–145.

Sano M, Ernesto MS, Thomas RG (1997) A controlled trial of Selegiline, alpha-tocopherol, or both as treatment for Alzheimer's disease. *N Engl J Med* **17:** 1216–1217.

Standing Medical Advisory Committee (1998) Advice 5/98 Donepezil for Alzheimer's Disease. London, UK: Department of Health.

Sim A (1999) Rivastigmine: a review. *Hospital Medicine* **60:** 731–735.

Teri L, Rabins P, Whitehouse P et al (1992) Management of behavior disturbance in Alzheimer's disease: current knowledge and future directions. *Alzheimer Dis Assoc Disord* **6:** 77–88.

Wilcock G (2000) Cognitive improvement in memantine in a placebo-controlled trial in mild to moderate vascular dementia. Sixth International Stockholm/Springfield Symposium on Advances in Alzheimer's Therapy 5–8 April.

chapter 5

Occupational therapy interventions

Ruth Chaplin

Occupation is that which we seize for our own possession, because it has meaning and value for us, habitually and fully engages our time, attention and environment.

(Perrin and May, 1999)

The aim of the occupational therapist (OT) is to enable people to live productive and enjoyable lives. We believe that activity is fundamental to well-being and we aim to restore function where performance of activity has been interrupted by ill health. This may be by helping the person to develop the adaptive skills required to maintain, restore or acquire function or by modifying an activity to maximize performance.

People are active and occupational by nature and these activities will be determined by their perceived roles and responsibilities and the influence of the culture and society in which they live. OTs believe that in order to maintain a state of well-being there should be a balance between the activities of self-care, productivity and leisure. Self-care is activity to maintain the individual such as washing, dressing, preparing and eating food. Productivity is activity to maintain the environment or to acquire sustenance such as preparing food for others, studying or doing paid or unpaid work. Leisure is activity to fulfil a person's own creative, aesthetic, physical and social needs such as hobbies and socializing (CAOT, 1997).

As a person grows older, the nature and balance of these activities may be expected to change gradually. However, for a person of working age diagnosed with a dementia this balance will be interrupted without warning. Their role within the family will change as will the roles of those around them and it will be difficult for all to adapt. The expectations, hopes and plans of the family will now have to be re-evaluated. The challenge for the OT is to maximize the skills and strengths of the person and his/her environment to enhance his/her quality of life.

This chapter will try to illustrate some of the main differences in working with younger people with dementia in contrast to experience gained with older people, while acknowledging the many similarities and common themes.

Following occupational therapy assessment (Chapter 3), the strengths and needs of the individuals and their current level of activity should be clear. They will also have identified which activities they value and are therefore motivated to perform. From this information the OT will be able to devise a plan of treatment in conjunction with each individual.

The aims of occupational therapy interventions with younger people with dementia

These aims can be summarized as follows; to:

- maximize and maintain functioning in activities of self-care, productivity and leisure.
- enhance self-esteem and confidence in the individual through the facilitation of appropriate activity.
- give advice and support to carers to enable them to maintain the individual's role within the home.
- work with other agencies to ensure that the person, and his/her carer if applicable, receive appropriate support in the home to maintain his/her well-being and safety.

- work with other agencies to ensure that the person has access to appropriate community facilities for adults.

The principles of occupational therapy interventions with younger people with dementia

Interventions should be:

- *Age-appropriate*. It is important to use activities that are appropriate to people's age and not to think of them as an older person because of their diagnosis or their level of impairment.
- *Culturally valued*. People's cultural context should be a part of any treatment plan and it is important to use activities that are culturally appropriate and that are seen as worthwhile and important by those around them.
- *Person-centred*. While all activities may not have been identified by the individuals, the OT should find out as much as he/she can about their likes and dislikes in order to plan treatment that is appropriate to them as individuals. As Turner (1997) says, 'Purposeful activity motivates a person to participate because it has meaning and is related to his goals'.
- *Achievable*. Failure in an activity is very detrimental to self-esteem and confidence and the activity should be analysed and adapted so that the OT knows the level of support needed to enable the individual to achieve the activity.
- *Productive and /or active*. This is very important in working with younger people with dementia. They are of working age and may recently have left paid employment. The pain of the loss of their working role may still be acute and with it the loss of status and self-esteem. Therefore, activities that have a good end-product that they can be proud of achieving are very valuable. Activities that incorporate physical exercise are also important as many of our

clients are physically very fit and active. However, our clients with Alzheimer's disease often have marked visuospatial deficits and dyspraxia and care must be taken to use activities that can be carried out by people of all abilities (e.g. horticultural activities or walks in the countryside).

Interventions in self-care activities

The OT will be aiming to maximize and maintain functioning in self-care activities. This will be done by analysing and adapting a task so that the person can achieve all or a part of that task. It will also be done by providing aids and adaptations to the environment to facilitate performance.

The loss of self-care skills in younger people can be very distressing both for the individuals and their carers. To have to assist your partner in dressing and intimate self-care tasks is very difficult at any stage in a relationship, and the clients and carers of our service have talked about the embarrassment and loss of dignity and self-esteem it engenders in a younger person. Our clients are sometimes very reluctant to accept any help in self-care tasks from outside agencies and we often have to be very involved in these areas. The therapeutic relationship between the OT and the clients and their carers is very important in this area of activity. It is often not appropriate or helpful to try to address these issues initially, but to build up a good working relationship based around leisure or productive activities. This ongoing relationship centred on positive activities then enables us to subsequently broach the area of self-care. This illustrates the need for early intervention and an ongoing relationship with clients and carers.

As with older people with dementia, analysis and adaptation of a task may help to promote independence in some part of the self-care activity. For example, people with a dressing dyspraxia may be able to put on their clothes if they are passed to them in the correct order and appropriate gestures given. People who are not able to coordinate their movements in using a knife and fork may be able to use a fork to eat food if it is cut up for them or if a carer initially gestures the pattern of movement. We have found it very useful to give such advice to carers in written form as well as demonstrating such techniques to them. The input of a speech and language therapist (Chapter 3) is also very useful in advising on strategies to enhance verbal and non-verbal communication in these areas of activity.

Aids and adaptations may be useful, for example, an insulated plate for someone who eats very slowly or a plate guard for someone who is having difficulty getting food on to his/her fork. Their use must be balanced with the risk of stigmatizing a person in their environment. It may be appropriate to make interventions in the structuring of a person's self-care activities where there has been a loss of role or motivation. An approach used in the Manchester Carisbrooke service is to agree on priorities of tasks, and then write down a plan to integrate these activities back into the individual's daily or weekly routine.

Interventions in productivity

The OT aims to maximize and maintain function in areas of productive activity. It is very important to establish where clients' interests and motivations lie and this will have been discussed during the assessment period (Chapter 3). For many of our clients, the loss of skills and confidence will have led to other members of their family taking tasks away from them. The OT will identify tasks or parts of tasks that the person is still able to do and give advice about the level of supervision needed. For example, the OT will advise on the use of memory aids, such as calendars and memo boards, to help the person to structure his/her productive activities. Advice can be given on aids to safety, such as smoke alarms, gas detectors or cooker isolation taps, to enable the person to continue to prepare food for his/her family and to continue to live in the community as safely as possible.

The loss of paid employment is a very emotive issue for our clients and their carers. Most of our clients have already left their employment when they come to us and all have stories to tell about how difficult it has been. Where they are still in employment, we work with employers to see if the client's role can be adapted and to plan for the cessation of employment when necessary (see Case study 1).

Unpaid or vocational employment should always be considered especially if the younger person's condition is stable (e.g. in a Korsakoff-type dementia). We have made referrals to work-orientated projects in the community such as woodworking or gardening projects. Sometimes, our clients are excluded because of their diagnosis and then our service takes an advocacy role, arguing for the opportunity for them to be assessed on their strengths and needs and not to be prejudiced by their diagnosis.

Case study 1

Catherine is 59 years old and has a diagnosis of Alzheimer's disease. She is single, has no children and is not in touch with any of her family. She has a slight learning disability and has never learnt to read or write fluently. At the time of referral to our service, Catherine was still working part-time as a cleaner in a local college. Her employer was aware that Catherine was not able to carry out her duties to the required standard and she and her colleagues had adapted her work tasks to their simplest level. Her employer felt that they were coming to a point where Catherine would have to retire on grounds of incapacity to work.

On assessment, it was found that Catherine's self-care skills were poor due to a lack of motivation and awareness rather than an inability to perform tasks. She lived in a very poorly maintained flat near to her work, which was on the top floor of a Victorian house, and she was struggling to get up and down the three flights of stairs. Catherine was having breakfast and lunch at her workplace and not preparing food at all in her flat.

All of Catherine's productive activities were centred around her workplace; she did not see anyone else but her work colleagues and spent the rest of her time alone in her flat. Following the completion of a leisure profile, Catherine expressed an interest in practising her literacy skills, which had never been very good, and she also said that she would like to try to learn how to swim. We arranged for her to attend a suitable literacy class where the tutor was aware that Catherine was attending the classes for enjoyment and social contact and may not progress in her learning. She also started attending a keep fit class for the over-50s that included a session in the pool in the afternoons when she had finished work. Catherine derived a lot of enjoyment from these new activities and when they were part of her weekly routine she was more open to discussing her retirement from work. We gradually reduced the number of days per week she was working and also arranged a day care place at a local day centre and home carer support with housework, bills and shopping.

Catherine retired nine months after our first contact and a month later moved into warden-controlled accommodation near to the day centre. Moving a person with a dementia into new accommodation is usually not recommended but we had little alternative in this case as Catherine's flat was unsuitable. After an intensive period of orientation into her new surroundings she settled well into the social life there and was able to maintain herself and her environment with a full package of care from Social Services and our Carisbrooke service.

Case study 2

Gary is 59 years old and has a diagnosis of Korsakoff syndrome and a past head injury. He also has depression and anxiety.

Gary lives with his second wife and their 13-year-old son. Both of them have grown-up families from their first marriages. Gary was employed as a builder and he provided well for his family. He can no longer work and his family has experienced financial hardship. He lacks confidence and self-esteem because he can no longer provide for his family.

Gary misses the camaraderie and physical challenge of working. Following assessment, it was clear that he still retained some of his physical skills and was able to concentrate on activities for short amounts of time. He found that his anxiety was reduced by being involved in an activity and that this lessened his negative thoughts. Gary did not feel that domestic activities were appropriate for him but he agreed to help his wife, who suffers from arthritis, with some heavier chores such as shopping.

Gary had a keen interest in gardening, having once had an allotment. This interest was harnessed to provide some structure both at home and in day care. At his home, we provided several small tomato plants with some compost. Gary's task was to pot them into growbags in his garden and to water and feed them on a daily basis, with some prompting from his wife. We also devised a plan of action so that he could gradually introduce other plants into the rest of his garden and take some responsibility for these. This was an activity that he could do with his son who is also interested in gardening and it became the focus of some very valuable time that they spent together each day. It helped his motivation, increased his levels of physical exercise and added structure to his day. It also increased his confidence and self-esteem in that he was able to achieve a task and get positive feedback for this. Gary also became very involved in the Allotment Project, described later in this chapter, and we continue to work with him to provide suitable horticultural activities all year round.

Leisure interventions

A leisure profile is completed with each person as part of the assessment process. The OT will look at adapting existing activities to the person's strengths by analysing the activity and what skills it requires. Depending on the outcome of assessment and the person's skills and motivations, it may be appropriate to look at new interests rather than concentrating on those previously held. For example, if someone has a love of painting or drawing but is no longer able to achieve good end-results in this activity, his/her creative interest can be adapted to activities, such as pottery or painting on silk, which require much less complex skills but in which good end-results are more easily achievable with appropriate support.

Prior to diagnosis, many younger people with dementia will have had a very good social life, their children will be grown up and they may have an income that provides a good standard of living. Some may be starting new relationships, planning towards retirement and looking forward to enjoying the benefits of their hard work. They may have very active leisure interests; playing football, metal detecting, golf and nature rambling are just a few of the interests of our clients.

New or existing leisure activities will need to be incorporated into the person's daily routine and we always try to include leisure activities that the person and his/her carer can do together. After diagnosis, carers are often very downhearted as they feel that all the pleasurable activities that they did with their loved one are affected and we try to give them support to adapt these activities rather than ceasing them altogether. For example, if a couple have enjoyed eating out or going out socially, this should continue but perhaps in quieter places or at quieter times, and with friends or family members who have some understanding of the illness. Holidays may have been an important part of a person and his/her family's life, and again we will give information and advice about possible hotels and organizations that are helpful and appropriate to that person's needs. We also have information about grants that are available to help with holiday costs and costs of leisure activities for the person and carer.

It may be appropriate to involve other statutory and voluntary agencies in enabling leisure activities. Often at the Carisbrooke service we recommend the involvement of local services. These include Adult Placement, in which a family unit offers supportive care in the family home and Crossroads Caring for Carers, a volunteer group that offers support. We also recommend befriending services and, recently, we have had access to a new service, the Admiral Nursing Service, in which the caregiver is the designated client. It is also important that younger people with dementia have access to leisure facilities in the local community. Other local services used with clients include library services, such as services for the visually impaired and internet access, leisure centres for swimming, keep fit sessions, gym facilities, and Adult Education Centres for leisure-based courses.

The Allotment Project

An activity that fits all of the principles and aims of interventions with younger people with dementia is horticulture. In Manchester, in addition to providing horticultural activities in the person's home and in day care centres we also have an allotment (Figure 5.1). We do not have any safe garden space in our day care setting and so we rent an allotment from a local allotment society at a cost of £28 per annum. The project has proved to be very beneficial for a whole range of our clients as it involves a variety of activities that are familiar and use normal patterns of movement. Its emphasis on productivity, fresh air

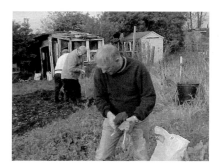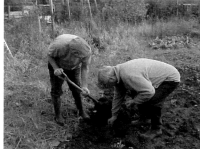

Figure 5.1 *The Carisbrooke allotment project.*

and exercise is particularly appropriate for our clients and it has the bonus of being in a peaceful and relaxing environment. The project is described in more detail in an article in the *Alzheimer's Society Newsletter* (Chaplin, 2000). Useful information on horticultural activities with people with dementia is also available from Thrive Publications (see the References for the address).

Interventions in the later stages of illness

Many of the above interventions are appropriate for the early to middle stages of dementia. In the later stages, all of the principles of intervention should still apply but there will need to be a re-evaluation of the needs of the person and his/her carer and a review of interventions. For some of our clients this may be a more intensive package of home care and for others it may mean a move to nursing home care. Continuity of input from our care team is very important and is something that carers have said has helped them through this very difficult time.

The role of life history books

Individuality means having continuity between your past, your present and your future.

King's Fund, 1988.

Life history books, such as *Memoraid* (see References) or memory diaries, are very useful in the later stages of a dementia. Ideally, they should be compiled gradually over a number of months with the participation of the person and his/her family and friends. They should contain important personal information such as life history, likes and dislikes, important people and all relevant contacts. Photographs are also very useful. This information is invaluable for other agencies involved with the client and is an important part of person-centred care.

References

CAOT (Canadian Association of Occupational Therapists) (1997) *Enabling Occupation; an Occupational Therapy Perspective.* Ottawa: CAOT publications.

Chaplin R (2000) Green Fingers. *Alzheimer's Society Newsletter.* **Dec:** 8.

King's Fund (1988) *Living Well into Old Age. Applying Principles of Practice to Services for People with Dementia.* London: King's Fund.

Perrin T, May H (2000) *Well Being in Dementia. An Occupational Approach for Therapists and Carers.* Edinburgh: Churchill Livingstone.

Memoraid (2001) 43 Brunswick Quay, Rotherhithe, London SE16 7PU.

Thrive Publications, Geoffrey Udall Centre, Beech Hill, Reading RG7 2AT.

Turner A, Foster M, Johnson S (1997) *Occupational Therapy and Physical Dysfunction.* Edinburgh: Churchill Livingstone, p 106.

chapter 6

Psychological interventions

Emma Shlosberg

Caregiver burden and the use of cholinesterase inhibitors have received the most attention and evaluation in the field of dementia care. However, the use of pharmacological treatments is not always appropriate and may not be effective for all clients. The introduction of psychosocial interventions for people with dementia is therefore timely as they can also be used in conjunction with, and subsequently to complement, pharmacological treatments.

The chapter comprises:

- An outline of the specific role of the clinical psychologist in the Carisbrooke (Manchester) service.
- An overview of the principles of working with younger people who have dementia.
- Discussion of the particular issues to consider when working with younger people with dementia.
- Consideration of engagement issues.
- Descriptions of specific psychological approaches.
- Discussion of clinical effectiveness and future directions.

Skills of the clinical psychologist

Clinical psychologists are health care professionals working predominantly in the field of mental health. Within the Manchester Younger Persons Dementia Service the role of the clinical psychologist primarily involves:

- *Psychological assessment.* A broad range of assessments are available, including behavioural assessment, assessment of mood and assessment to assist in defining a strengths/needs profile of cognitive function. All of these assessment techniques allow the clinician to gain a better understanding of the presenting problem.
- *Psychological intervention.* This is the use of psychological methods of proven effectiveness in helping others bring about change. Interventions take place not only with the person with dementia, but also with families and those services that support the person.
- *Psychological evaluation.* Not only on a case-by-case basis but also to objectively evaluate the impact of new and emerging services such as the Carisbrooke service.
- *Consultancy work/Staff liaison.*
- *Teaching/Training.*
- *Research.*

Principles of working with younger people with dementia

The pioneering work of Kitwood (1997) has shifted the focus of dementia care from viewing neurological impairment as the most important influence on the dementing process to viewing people with dementia as unique individuals each with their own personalities, biographies and emotions. Kitwood argues that the environment and the social interactions within it (i.e. social psychology) can play a part in destroying the 'personhood' of the person with dementia. This has been termed 'malignant social psychology' and is a concept used to explain practices that serve to disempower and devalue people with dementia. This work has resulted in the emergence of 'a new culture of dementia care' of which a crucial aspect concerns maintaining personhood by recognizing that each individual has unique needs, preferences, likes, dislikes, fears and anxieties. This new culture of care encourages carers to be more empathic and consider the subjective experience of dementia.

As with those with older age dementia, each younger person with dementia is a unique individual with a different life history and needs. The gold standard is to implement an individually tailored approach that will vary depending on the type of dementia, the stage of acceptance, availability of support networks, the stage of illness, individual life histories, coping mechanisms and social situation.

Issues to consider when working with younger people with dementia

Historically, people with dementia have been a disempowered and devalued group of individuals. Working with younger people who have dementia may therefore raise a number of professional and therapeutic challenges that will need to be addressed in clinical supervision. In particular:

- Attention needs to be paid to the dynamic of the therapist/patient relationship ensuring that the person with dementia is being listened to and that power issues are acknowledged and kept to a minimum.
- The personal impact of such work requires consideration. The work may evoke deep emotional reactions due to the nature and complexity of problems that some individuals may bring.
- The emergence of counter transference, as in the therapist experiencing feelings towards the patient (client) that link to the therapist's own past.

- Risks of over-identification due to perceived commonality ('I would feel like that in your shoes'). The therapist therefore needs to be alert to the possibility of projecting his/her feelings and anxieties on to the person with young onset dementia.
- The work may require multidisciplinary liaison (e.g. HIV liaison, home carers, etc.), and with it, competence at consulting with other disciplines.
- Acceptance that the person's cognitive abilities may deteriorate over the course of therapy. This may require flexibility and creativity on the part of the therapist.
- Insight into the degree of retained cognitive abilities, with a view to building on these to maximize self-esteem and quality of life.
- Awareness of premorbid coping styles. Caution should be exercised when engaging in such work as it may cause increased insight into deficits. Therefore, careful consideration should be given as to how the individual is likely to react before embarking thereon.
- Knowledge of available support networks.
- The therapy goals should be individually tailored, achievable, measurable, monitored and agreed. In some cases, there may be a need for graded task assignment that involves breaking goals down into smaller, more achievable, mini goals.
- Realization that short-term gains may be a more realistic outcome due to the progressive nature of dementia.

Engagement issues

The following points may assist in maximizing appropriate engagement in therapy:

- Have shorter, more frequent, therapy sessions.
- Provide written summaries of session contents or tape-record sessions.

- Offer regular feedback and repetition in session.
- Provide breaks in sessions.
- Consider the pace, which may need to be much slower.
- Work with carers allowing them to act as co-therapists between treatment sessions.
- Set realistic goals and foster realistic hope.
- Avoid the use of jargon and abstract phrases.
- Use audio and/or video tapes to compensate for memory difficulties.
- Be flexible, particularly in relation to the location of therapy.

Individual approaches

The list below is by no means exhaustive and unfortunately a detailed description of all therapeutic techniques is beyond the scope of this chapter. An overview of those interventions most commonly practised in the Carisbrooke service is therefore presented.

Dealing with losses

Historically, sharing diagnoses with people suffering from dementia rarely occurred. Reasons included fear of catastrophic psychological effects, a belief that nothing could be done, uncertainty surrounding the diagnosis, or a belief that the individual would not understand, so 'why bother'. Although withholding diagnosis may be appropriate in some instances of severe cognitive impairment, it does not apply to those individuals who retain insight and want to better understand their experiences. There is now a general consensus that such information should be shared with the person affected as it will enable financial matters to be organized and issues relevant to driving ability to be addressed. It may also assist in access to appropriate treatments (both psychological and pharmacological); it may facilitate appropriate adjustment for both sufferer and family alike and is more likely to provide a framework within which the person affected and family members can understand their experiences.

Best practice involves:

■ The professional gaining insight into what the individual has already been told.
■ A clear and early diagnosis framed in a way that can be easily understood.
■ Consideration of how the information will be shared.
■ Consideration of what and how to disclose the information
■ Sensitivity, discretion and flexibility.
■ Follow-up: sharing the diagnosis should not be a one-off event but rather a dynamic and evolving process.

Providing a forum for people with dementia to express and vent their feelings following diagnosis is essential. Issues related to losses will invariably be raised and the therapist's role is to provide conditions in which appropriate grieving can occur. Many younger individuals with dementia retain insight into their condition and may encounter difficulties accepting the cognitive and/or physical changes. A variety of cognitive and emotional responses including shock or disbelief, distress and depression, frustration, anger, withdrawal and isolation may emerge but if these are vented in a supportive forum, appropriate adjustment is more likely to occur.

Memory rehabilitation

The main aims of memory rehabilitation are to:

■ Optimize functioning.
■ Utilize preserved abilities.
■ Increase self-esteem and well-being.
■ Prevent a pattern of excess disability where the person functions less well than expected relative to the degree of cognitive impairment.
■ Develop new resources to cope with cognitive difficulties.

If rehabilitation programmes are to be effective, it is important to carry out a detailed assessment of cognitive functioning. Not only will this provide a baseline but it will also allow for a deeper understanding of the individual's areas of strength and the extent and degree of impairment. Just as important is close multidisciplinary liaison that will allow pooling of qualitative information about the individual's strengths, areas of need and personality. Such liaison will also allow appropriate and realistic goal-setting to occur. The importance of the environment or social situation must not be underestimated. An environment that is encouraging and stimulating will maximize the chances of success. Other characteristics that are important in achieving performance gains are an adequate (often long) training period, approaches that involve caregivers and the use of training strategies that are based on well-preserved abilities (Godley and Gatz, 2000).

Examples of memory rehabilitation techniques include:

1   *Assisting individuals in learning and retaining small amounts of relevant information.*

   ■ Expanded rehearsal (Camp and Stevens, 1990) involves adjusting the retrieval period during learning, one item at a time, according to whether the item was successfully recalled on the earlier trial. If the item was successfully recalled, the retrieval period is doubled; if not recalled successfully, the retrieval period is halved. This process is continued until the information is recalled after the desired interval. Such techniques have been used, successfully, to teach names of common objects and to enhance prospective memory performance. However, Woods (1994) believes the effort required may exceed the gains achieved and recommends its use with items that affect quality of life.

   ■ Errorless learning (Wilson et al, 1994) is a technique that ensures that frank errors—which may get encoded and remembered—are avoided when information is being encoded. This involves discouraging the need to guess by ensuring successful encoding at each stage.

93

2 *Encouragement in the use of external memory aides.* Such environmental adaptations and aides aim to reduce the demands on memory. The use of diaries or memory wallets, one page a day calendars, checklists and notebooks, can all be used to minimize demands on orientation and memory for relevant personal information. However, these techniques may need to be supplemented by regular prompts by carers to ensure the habit of utilizing such aides is developed. Positive outcomes have been reported with such techniques (e.g. improved conversational ability), in terms of quality and quantity.

3 *Building on preserved memory abilities, often memory for skills, or factual information.*

Validation therapy

Feil (1993) suggested that certain features associated with dementia, such as the tendency for individuals to retreat into the past, are ways for the individual to avoid distress, loneliness and boredom. It is suggested that the reality of having dementia is too painful and so individuals withdraw into a 'fantasy' world. Validation therapy emphasizes the emotional world of the person with dementia and attempts are made to validate their feelings, thus allowing individuals to move from their inner world into the shared reality of the present. The technique proposes empathic listening, acceptance and warmth, and aims to make the individual feel understood and accepted.

This therapy encourages individuals to look beyond the words spoken and explore the hidden meanings and feelings behind them in an attempt to understand the person and his/her current feelings and emotions. In this way, these techniques may assist in restoring a sense of emotional well-being. Hitch (1994) suggested that they could result in less negative affect, promote social interaction and may reduce the occurrence of behavioural disturbance. However, a number of authors have emphasized the importance of exercising caution with this technique and not to overlook an individual's attempt to communicate basic needs by focusing too much on confused conversation.

Tips to help communication include:

- Eliminating distractions (e.g. television, radio).
- Ensuring the person can see and hear you.
- Maintaining eye contact.
- Identifying yourself by name even if you are well known.
- Simplifying and shortening sentences.
- Using non-verbal cues such as nods and gestures. Gentle touch can also reinforce your presence.
- Speaking slowly and clearly.
- Encouraging discussion of topics of interest to the person with dementia.
- Being a good listener.
- Not rushing but taking your time.

Cognitive behaviour therapy (CBT)

CBT highlights the association between thoughts, feelings and behaviour and has been used on a limited scale for individuals with mild cognitive impairment. It can be used to treat, amongst others, depression, anxiety, shame and distress (Ballard et al, 2001). Those individuals with advanced young onset dementia may benefit from a more behavioural focus, whereas cognitive approaches are more appropriate for early stage dementia (Teri and Gallagher-Thompson, 1991).

Beck (1976), one of the pioneers of cognitive therapy, suggests that mood is influenced by the occurrence of automatic (because they pop into awareness) negative thoughts and images. Using depression as an example Beck introduced the idea of a cognitive triad whereby an individual's negative thoughts centre around the three areas shown in Figure 6.1

The tendency to view situations negatively is due to a number of thinking errors such as:

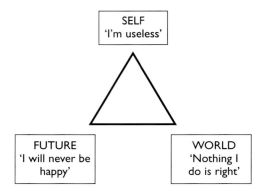

Figure 6.1 *A cognitive triad.*

- *Overgeneralization*: making sweeping judgements based on single instances.
- *Selective abstraction*: attending to the negative aspects of experiences.
- *Dichotomous reasoning*: thinking in extremes (i.e. black-and-white thinking).
- *Personalization*: taking responsibility for things that have little or nothing to do with oneself.

During an episode of depression these negative thoughts appear credible and an individual's ability to consider more plausible or realistic alternative thoughts is greatly diminished.

CBT aims to assist individuals by:

1 Implementing behavioural strategies that allow individuals to re-engage in activities that evoke feelings of pleasure and/or mastery. These techniques are aimed at stimulating individuals to use and maintain their residual cognitive and social abilities.

2 Providing strategies that assist individuals in identifying and challenging their negative thought patterns, enabling more plausible and objective thinking patterns to emerge. A complicating factor is that in the case of a younger person with dementia some of the negative thoughts may be realistic. It is therefore important to make

the distinction between the actual and perceived negative thoughts. The negative thoughts and feelings can be documented by the use of simplified diaries.

However, it is important to mention that not everyone responds favourably to the use of diaries. The identification of thoughts therefore may need to take place in session time.

Once the problem has been conceptually understood a number of strategies are proposed such as:

- Listing the advantages and disadvantages of this style of thinking.
- Examining the evidence for and against specific thoughts.
- Considering whether the client is adopting certain thinking styles such as jumping to conclusions based on insufficient evidence.

Successful CBT hinges on a collaborative relationship between patient and therapist and, in order to facilitate this process, regular sessions are advised which will also assist in fostering feelings of security and familiarity.

Most of the available outcome studies use a behavioural approach focused on the treatment of depression. Positive results, such as increasing the frequency and duration of pleasant activities, improvements in mood and decreased occurrence of 'troublesome' behaviours, have been reported.

Case study 1

Brian, a middle-aged man, was initially referred to the clinical psychology services for neuropsychological testing. Results suggested a patchy pattern of cognitive impairment in keeping with alcohol-related dementia. Concerns were raised about Brian's mood state. Therefore, following completion of the assessment a course of CBT was recommended.

Following detailed psychosocial assessment it emerged that Brian was suffering from episodes of low mood characterized by spells of isolation and withdrawal, negative styles of thinking and reduced confidence. Although Brian previously coped with difficulties by drinking alcohol he had stopped drinking since receiving his diagnosis and this left him without a mechanism to cope with the assorted losses in his life (cognitive functioning, family contact, status, finances, etc.).

Brian was asked to record his weekly activities. Examination revealed that, with the exception of day care, Brian was engaging in no meaningful or enjoyable activities. Activities that

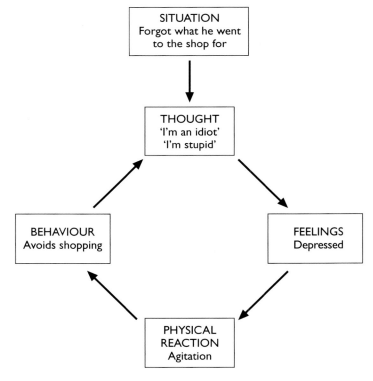

Figure 6.2 *Case study 1: mini formulation of negative thoughts.*

evoked feelings of pleasure or mastery were collaboratively generated and Brian was encouraged to begin incorporating them into his weekly timetable.

Brian was also asked to record those situations that caused distress and the accompanying negative thoughts in a simplified diary. One example is depicted in the mini formulation shown in Figure 6.2.

After a number of weeks thought re-evaluation techniques were introduced in session (and in a handout format) that allowed more objective styles of thinking to emerge.

Considering the nature of cognitive impairment the therapist also felt it necessary to build on Brian's strengths. He clearly had a number of retained cognitive abilities and it was envisaged that by building on these preserved abilities this would also serve to increase his self-esteem, independence and quality of life.

Behaviour modification

A common referral to a clinical psychologist requests assessment of various 'challenging behaviours'. These behaviours can heighten feelings of caregiver burden and may result in institutionalization and/or maladaptive practices such as physical restraint or over-medication.

When working in the field of dementia care the use of pejorative terms such as 'attention-seeker', 'violent', or 'disruptive' is unfortunately all too common. Stokes (1995) argues for the formulation of an operational definition in collaboration with the care team. This technique advocates the use of unambiguous terms enabling detailed descriptions of behaviours that leave little room for misunderstanding.

Behaviour modification aims to change patients' behaviours with techniques based on learning theory. Detailed assessment and good history-taking is essential and may involve meetings with family members or friends in order to gather detailed information about the

Table 6.1 ABC analysis

Date/Time	A	B	C	Background
	What were they doing *immediately before* the behaviour occurred? Who was there / wasn't there?	Describe precisely *what happened.* Where did it occur? What did the person do?	What happened *immediately after* the incident? How did others respond?	Has anything happened during the day to cause distress? Has there been change in routine?

individual's social, educational, occupational and life history, their personality, environmental issues, and exploration of any unmet needs.

Detailed observations often prove to be an invaluable source of information-gathering and knowledge can be gained about how others treat the person with dementia. Indeed, observations may also clarify those for whom behaviours are problematic. Has the referral been requested for staff convenience rather than patient benefit?

Most staff involved in dementia care are familiar with behavioural analysis (or ABC analysis) which allows exploration of 'A' activating or precipitating events, 'B' detailed description of the problem behaviour, and 'C' the consequences of that behaviour. Such information is usually recorded in a chart similar to the one depicted in Table 6.1.

It is important to gain baseline recordings over a period of about two weeks in order to determine a pattern. Regardless of the intervention, recording should continue to enable the frequency of the behaviours to be monitored.

Functional analysis is a more detailed form of descriptive analysis that provides understanding of a person's behaviour from a more holistic and person-centred perspective. It attempts to gain an understanding of the meaning and possible functions of behaviours. It looks beyond the simple ABC analysis and, in keeping with person-centred approaches, explores the intrapsychic (e.g. emotional) factors that are not observable. Information that can be gathered includes:

- brief patient description,
- family details,
- ecological analysis (i.e. description of the living environment; characteristics of family, residents or staff),
- schedule of activities including details as to whether they are age-appropriate and/or functional,
- health and medical status,
- current and past history of medication,
- previous treatment history,
- methods of communication including expressive and receptive language skills,
- cognitive abilities,
- activities of daily living,
- emotional issues,
- social skills.

Following the detailed analysis a number of hypotheses regarding the establishment and maintenance of the behaviour need to be generated. Possibly, the most crucial stage of functional analysis is the 'testing out' phase. This may involve close liaison with, and possibly some level of education for, those staff members unfamiliar with the techniques. It is important to remember that psychological contact does not cease upon completion of the assessment. It is an ongoing and evolving process that involves testing hypotheses and possibly reformulating the problem until the desired outcome is achieved.

In general, behavioural interventions are associated with reductions in the overall level of behavioural disturbance.

Case study 2

Lenny was referred for behavioural assessment by staff in a residential home. The referral requested assessment of a number of behavioural problems including:

1 Continually mimicking chewing.
2 Daily biting and scratching of staff. The behaviour was precipitated whenever staff attended to his care.

Staff tended to cope with the behaviours by either ignoring them or operating a number of safety behaviours to prevent injury. Lenny has a diagnosis of vascular dementia and is an insulin-dependent diabetic. He is registered blind, is wheelchair-bound and prone to constipation. Lenny has not communicated for several months and is totally dependent on staff for self-care.

The relevant background information was gathered from friends. Lenny was described as 'an intelligent and independent man' who enjoyed his own company. One of his few passions in life was to eat, to the extent that he had two fridges in his house and literally spent most of his days eating. Since his admission into long-term care Lenny had lost 9 stone (he previously weighed 18 stone). Staff referred to Lenny by his forename but discussions with the family revealed he only ever responded to a nickname.

Detailed observations were carried out. It emerged that staff would attend to Lenny's self-care without any prior warning (e.g. staff approaching Lenny from behind and administering his insulin without warning him first).

Impressions and analysis of meaning

Chewing:
■ This may be a direct attempt to communicate an unmet need—either hunger or pain.

■ Lenny's previous dietary habits and love of food suggest that the chewing may be a lifetime habit.

Biting and scratching:

■ Lenny may have been alarmed. Observations revealed episodes where staff approached Lenny from behind or engaged in contact without any warning. Considering Lenny's visual impairment, unexplained or rapid approaches by staff were likely to evoke a hostile act of self-protection. To compound the problem, staff members referred to Lenny by an unfamiliar name.

■ Lenny may have a degree of insight into his cognitive difficulties. Attempts to assist with self-care may be unwelcome, particularly when considering his premorbid personality.

A number of recommendations were made including:
— The staff calling Lenny the name he is used to.
— Referral to the dietician to explore the possibility of increasing his dietary intake.
— Exploring ways to increase Lenny's quality of life.
— Ensuring that staff members approach Lenny in a gentle and non-confrontational manner and warn him when they are about to attend to his self-care.
— Exploring the possibility that Lenny was in pain.

Clinical effectiveness

The difficulty of measuring outcome in dementia care may explain the paucity of available outcome studies. Outcome studies that are available are often riddled with methodological flaws meaning the generalizability effects are unknown. There are some qualitative evaluation studies that are largely unconvincing. Perhaps future work could make use of a single case methodology to focus on the reduction of challenging behaviours as a way of measuring effectiveness or, in keeping with the new models of dementia care, perhaps another way would be to evaluate levels of 'well-being' (humour, initiating social interaction, etc.).

Future directions

Although there are pockets of excellent dementia care, the concept of offering psychotherapeutic interventions to people with dementia continues to be a relatively new idea. For this reason, work in this field may need to be initiated by the individual clinician rather than relying on receiving direct referrals. This may also create a niche for educating other professionals and familiarizing them with a model of person-centred approaches. Theoretically, all people with dementia could potentially benefit from psychotherapy if the primary aim is to facilitate individuals in making sense of their own experiences of having dementia, that is, offering emotional support.

Although most work has been carried out with older people with dementia, there appears to be no reason why these techniques cannot be applied to younger people with dementia. Generally, within the field of dementia care, attitudes and the way people view dementia need to change. Older styles of thinking, that a person behaves in a certain way 'because of their dementia', need to be replaced with more person-centred approaches. This calls for more research focusing specifically on younger people, increased training opportunities for professionals and more positive images of dementia and dementia care for lay people.

References

Ballard CG, O'Brien J, James I, Swann A (2001) *Dementia: Management of Behavioural and Psychological symptoms.* Oxford: Oxford University Press.

Beck AT (1976) *Cognitive Therapy and the Emotional Disorders.* New York: International University Press.

Camp CJ, Stevens AB (1990) Spaced retrieval: a memory intervention for dementia of the Alzheimer's type (DAT). *Clin Gerontologist* **10:** 58–61.

Feil N (1993) *The Validation Breakthrough: Simple Techniques for Communicating with People with Alzheimer's type Dementia.* Baltimore: Health Profession's Press.

Godley K, Gatz M (2000) Psychosocial interventions for individuals with dementia: an integration of theory, therapy and a clinical understanding of dementia. *Clin Psychol Rev* **20:** 755–782.

Hitch S (1994) Cognitive therapy as a tool for the caring elderly confused person. *J Clin Nurs* **3:** 49–55.

Kitwood T (1997) *Dementia Reconsidered: the Person Comes First.* Buckingham: Open University Press.

Stokes G (1995) Incontinent or not? Don't label: Describe and assess. *J Dementia Care* **3:** 20–21.

Teri L, Gallagher-Thompson D (1991) Cognitive behavioural interventions for treatment of depression in Alzheimer's patients. *Gerontologist* **31:** 413–416.

Wilson BA, Baddeley A, Evans JJ et al (1994) Errorless learning in the rehabilitation of memory impaired people. *Neuropsychol Rehabil* **4:** 307–326.

Woods B (1994) Management of memory impairment in older people with dementia. *Int Rev Psychiatry* **6:** 153–161.

chapter 7

Social worker and social care: Roles and interventions

Sally Mendham

Roles

In England, the role of social services departments and social workers has seen some marked changes of emphasis since the NHS and Community Care Act 1990. The welcome move towards more community-based services has been tempered by increasing demand on limited resources brought about by earlier hospital discharges, a growing elderly population and increasing life expectancy. At the same time, the quest for visible public accountability and charging policies has led to an emphasis on the more measurable 'hands on' physical aspects of care and keeping labour costs to a minimum. In dealing with younger people with dementia, however, traditional social work skills as well as care management are needed. A person-centred approach, as originally outlined in the work of Tom Kitwood (1997) (also discussed in Chapter 6), is essential. He demonstrated how the disability from dementing illnesses cannot just be seen in the light of neurological impairment but also by unmet social, emotional, physical, psychological and spiritual needs. We all have needs for attachment, occupation, comfort, identity and inclusion. The way these are met in younger people who develop dementing illnesses, particularly in those also who have rarer conditions, will often differ from their older counterparts. Expectations of, and interactions with, younger people in general are not the same as those of older people who have retired, have grown families and differing responsibilities. This difference in needs is reflected in the needs of those with dementia and requires a specialist approach by the social worker (SW). This can be demonstrated by examining the skills and knowledge required of a SW in this field and exploring how they translate into interventions.

Skills (Table 7.1)

The SW's assessment may aid diagnosis, and/or facilitate the construction of an appropriate care plan. In England, at the time of writing, single assessment processes are being developed across primary care and social services. It is not yet clear what their format will be but it is likely that there will be a general information section with room for additional specialist recording. If done well this could enable quicker referral to appropriate services should there be a well-publicized single-referral pathway for younger people with dementia. The SW not only requires interviewing skills, based on specialist knowledge of the conditions involved and their impact, but also the ability to assess skills, ability and disability through engaging in activities with the person, especially if he/she is active. For example, a trip to the shops could highlight social skills, road sense, orientation, memory and money skills. An attempt to reduce assessment to tick boxes would be counter-productive.

The SW's initial contact is vital in establishing a supportive relationship; asking the right questions, openness, showing empathy, and knowledge of what may be helpful encourages trust. A pre-arranged visit at home, at a time arranged in consultation with all those involved, is likely to be the least stressful and provide valuable information towards assessment.

Depending on the composition of the core team, the SW's role may

Table 7.1 Skills of the social worker

- Interviewing and assessment
- Communication
- Care planning and monitoring
- Counselling and support; individual, family and group
- Multidisciplinary working
- Advocacy
- Networking
- Information and advice
- Training
- Ability to work alone in a challenging area

overlap in the area of assessment (Chapter 3). In the assessment the SW will be examining, with the person with dementia and family members, the following areas to determine need:

- personal, family, health and work history of the person,
- personality, interests, likes and dislikes,
- how the illness affects the person and others,
- family structure and relationships,
- sexuality,
- cultural issues,
- existing support networks,
- any areas of risk,
- financial situation and benefits entitlement,
- communication and language,
- the views of the person with dementia regarding his/her, and others' needs,
- the views of family members as to needs.

Communication skills are key to this process. Where a dementia may affect the communication process the SW needs to recognize this and make adjustments to the way he/she communicates. Listening, in the broadest sense of taking account of non-verbal as well as verbal communication, and checking understanding is an important part of this. The assessment should provide a picture of what the person with dementia may be experiencing and how this affects all around him/her; this requires the worker to empathize with him/her.

In England, carers have a right to a separate assessment under the Carers (Recognition and Services) Act 1995. The Carers' and Disabled Children's Act 2000 reinforces this right even when the cared-for person refuses assessment. This ensures that their needs are also considered; this may help in raising the priority for services and is particularly important in situations where there may be a conflict of interests. Included in 'carers' should be children and younger members of the family who may also find themselves in a caring situation, or in need of separate information and services. One example of service provision where this need has been acknowledged is Stockport Signpost for Carers (Greater Manchester), a local volunteer group, which runs a group for carers under the age of 18, where the emphasis is on shared activities with opportunity to talk about caring if wished. They would like to extend this service to 18- to 25-year-olds.

Assessment is a continuous process and the initial care plan should be adapted as the person with dementia, family members and the SW establish relationships and as the progression of the illness leads to changing needs. This highlights the importance of continuity of personnel involved in the care plan, repeated by families many times and mentioned in reports on provision for younger people with dementia, for example, The *Care Must be There* (Quinn, 1996); *Heading for Better Care* (NHSAS, 1996; Harvey, 1998). The alternative 'crisis management' approach is likely to lead to poorer quality of life and earlier admission to care.

Good multidisciplinary working entails good communication and an awareness of team members' roles and specific skills, with flexibility in areas of overlap. Thus, although other members of the team may use counselling and support skills, these are areas in which the SW is often involved. Information, practical advice and recognition of feelings, such as loss and isolation, can help begin the journey of learning to live with the illness. Where possible, knowledge of why, what, how and when things may happen and where to go for help can give back some feelings of control and can prevent extra stress caused by the feelings of uncertainty. Family members attending information/training groups in which the Stockport Dementia Care Training Project has been involved have confirmed this. Other examples are documented elsewhere in this book.

Financial, legal and work issues need to be examined. Having an early diagnosis allows planning for the future. The SW needs networking skills to help with planning and to advocate for the best available services for his/her client.

The focus of work may be on the person with dementia and/or family members. Family support is integral to the social work role. Families have to adapt to an illness in younger people which is often associated with older age and to changed roles. Due to the relative rarity of the situation, family members, child and adult, lack peer support and the SW can fulfil this role. SWs may be involved in family therapy (Chapter 11) and specialist support groups (Chapter 10). There may be occasions where conflict between family and the person with dementia would also lend itself to joint working between two members of the team or the involvement of an independent advocate.

Commissioning and introducing appropriate services needs sensitive handling: in the absence of age-appropriate services resistance to usage is particularly understandable. When commissioning non-specialist services the SW can have a training role with service providers, often needing to work alongside them to enable the necessary change in approach to working with younger, rather than older, people with dementia. Care plans (Chapter 3) should include a clear picture of the person, his/her likes and dislikes, and his/her strengths as well as weaknesses. In times of scarce resources arguing a priority need for services tends to encourage emphasis on the negative aspects of disability, but knowledge of an individual's abilities are vital for a workable care plan.

Good knowledge of the person and being able to see from his/her perspective makes it easier to avoid difficulties. However, determination to try again, perhaps with a different approach or with gradual introductions, is also important. A flexible, individual, needs-led approach is vital in working with younger people with dementia. Knowing how to do this within existing health and social care systems outside of specialist services, especially where charging policies are involved, can require considerable skill, knowledge, persistence and commitment. This leads on to consideration of other areas of knowledge necessary for the SW.

Knowledge (Table 7.2)

Social work skills should be based on knowledge of how particular dementias are likely to affect individuals and families in the short and long term, as well as the person-centred approach mentioned at the beginning of this chapter.

Having assessed the needs, the SW requires a good knowledge of suitable local and national resources and how to access them. A clear system of storing and updating such information is an invaluable tool. Included in this would be not only specialist services but also other

Table 7.2 Social work knowledge

- The referral path for medical assessment and diagnosis
- Disease processes and how these affect individuals and their carers
- Psychosocial model of understanding the disability caused and how best to enable the person
- Knowledge of effects of caring, likely carer needs and how best to enable carers
- Local and national resources and how to access them
- Welfare benefits
- Relevant legal and financial knowledge
- Broader-based social work knowledge for multiple social problem situations

non-specialist services that could meet needs with suitable support and information from the SW and/or other team members. Direct payment schemes may also be available locally. Personal contacts and first-hand experience of services enable suitable choices to be made and clearer lines of communication to be opened and maintained.

In addition to contacts with direct service providers, also important are those contacts involved in benefits, legal, financial and work issues. For instance, negotiations may need to be undertaken over pension rights or sickness payments following diagnosis. Financial issues are likely to be important in the current economic climate where mortgages require the contribution of two wage-earners. As well as the loss of income from the person with dementia, the partner taking on the role of carer can add additional strain. Early discussion of Enduring Powers of Attorney, wills and Advance Directives may help the person feel he/she has more control over what is happening as well as preventing possible future problems. Thus, the SW will need to know how to access specialist advice and have established working links. Knowledge of local solicitors who specialize in working with people with dementing illnesses and their relatives could be useful. In Britain, the Alzheimer's Society keeps a list of such solicitors, called Lawnet (Appendix 2). Likewise, links should be established with those who can give more in-depth welfare benefits advice over and above basic Disability Living Allowance, Invalid Care Allowance and Council Tax Rebates and deal with appeals where necessary.

Theory into practice: Specialist or not?

Case Study

Mrs Smith was 62 when referred to Social Services. She had a history of depression, and had been given a diagnosis of Alzheimer's disease by a general psychiatrist when in her mid-50s. There were no clear support structures at the time of diagnosis and she received no follow-up. What she and her family learnt was from local libraries. Her husband's diagnosis of a terminal illness eventually prompted the referral. After a basic assessment of needs and benefits check, services offered focused entirely on physical needs. Mrs Smith refused these and her husband continued his caring role. The case was closed.

Two weeks later her daughter had persuaded Mrs Smith to try a weekly support worker visit, which succeeded after a careful introduction. Mrs Smith may have had difficulty understanding fully when first asked: sometimes giving a concrete choice by trying something can be more meaningful than an abstract verbal decision. More time, and explanation, can also be helpful. The case was again closed.

Comment

The fact that there was no specific referral system for younger people with dementia meant that Mrs Smith and her family did not receive relevant information and advice following the diagnosis, nor were they put into contact with other services that might help; the networks were not there. The opportunity for using this early period to gather more information about Mrs Smith's past history, strengths, likes and dislikes and family situation and offer more emotional support was missed. A specialist worker could have made a considerable difference at this early stage.

The situation became a crisis when Mr Smith's death was imminent, introducing the danger that sudden decisions could be made for Mrs Smith rather than with her. A different SW allocated to the case saw Mr Smith, in hospital, once before he died. He reassessed Mrs Smith's capabilities, background information and caring needs. Finances and family situations were discussed openly; Mr Smith had already been planning ahead. Present and future plans were discussed. Time was spent enabling the SW and Mrs Smith to get to know each other so that emotional and physical support could be offered. The two daughters and son were anxious about their mother and wished to fulfil the wishes of their late father by ensuring she was looked after. The son felt that his mother should move in with him and his wife. The SW outlined the risks attached to further changes for Mrs Smith in discussions with the family, and when Mrs Smith clearly expressed her wish to remain at home, it was agreed that the care plan should support this.

The care plan was drawn up on the understanding that this could be amended as and when all involved, family and professionals, understood the situation better. The general practitioner was approached about a referral to an old age psychiatrist for a reassessment and, at the family's request, opinion about introducing cholinesterase inhibitors; also an occupational therapy assessment was sought. A communication book in the house, and Mrs Smith's own calendar ensured all involved knew what each other was doing. Much time was spent communicating with the family members, two of whom lived some distance away, but still visited regularly. Time was also allowed, in regular home visits, for the SW to discuss Mrs Smith's illness with her, allow her to voice her fears and her preferences for future care. The Alzheimer's Society booklet *So I have Dementia...* proved helpful. The SW, colleagues and family, were able to share observations of how Mrs Smith was managing and discuss ways to maintain skills with her. She continued going dancing, listening to music, watching videos and self-selected TV programmes. The care worker heated meals, one daughter ensured bathing during weekend visits and both helped with cleaning.

Comment

The SW at this stage had more involvement with Mrs Smith and took on the 'key worker' role, monitoring the care plan and assuming main responsibility for facilitating communication between all parties.

*By this time, an Old Age Psychiatry service had been estab-
lished in the area. Although not specializing in the management
of younger people with dementia, it retained health professionals
who had a particular interest in younger people with dementia
including a SW, and some of her social service colleagues. Thus
they worked as a multidisciplinary team and have since become
involved in pressing the case for increased provision. The
experience of other areas has demonstrated how pockets of
enthusiasm can provide the persistent pressure and publicity
necessary to ensure that the case for services for younger people
with dementia is heard. One example is that of Kensington and
Chelsea (London) where the pressure of some local families led to
the report 'The Care Must be There' (Quinn 1996), highlighting
the need for specialist services and professionals. Admiral nurses
(nurses whose clients are caregivers) were already working in
this area. The local authority funded a specialist day care service
for younger people with dementia and an action group was
formed. A few years later saw the opening of a specialist residential 10-bed unit within a nursing home for older people. A specialist SW was appointed who is based with other social work
colleagues. A combination of specialist younger people and
mainstream dementia services for older people is beginning to
work well because of a willingness of staff to be flexible to meet
the needs of younger people.*

To return to the case study, a number of concerns were voiced
by family and care workers. Mrs Smith went frequently to the
shops but no longer understood the value of money and could
forget to pay; her daughter was also worried about her crossing
roads. There were concerns about her poor nutritional intake
and being very choosy about food. The family also worried
about security as Mrs Smith hung her door key in an unlocked
outside cupboard when she went out. Risk assessments were
made and shared with all those involved, and the care plan

changed to minimize risks but preserve quality of life. When the SW learnt, through his networks, of a new specialist service in the neighbouring health authority, permission was sought to use this. Health and Social Services supported this and the psychiatrists involved liaised over medical details. Gradual introduction, through outreach, led to day care, where Mrs Smith appreciated age-appropriate meaningful activity, the sharing of problems by patients and the continuity of care provided by experienced staff. Once this was established, Mrs Smith accepted attendance at a voluntary-run local weekend day care service, where she enjoyed music and individual attention along with many older users who had dementia.

Comment

The importance of thorough, multidisciplinary risk assessments involving the family and the client is demonstrated. Extra services were needed as a result and it was through good networking and flexibility of approach that suitable provision was found. 'Out-of-area' services can be an extra burden for families, although in this case it was as close as local, but less appropriate, provision. Subsequently, however, such opportunities were discontinued due to the growth of local demand for the service.

The specialist service was preferable in meeting her needs, but the person-centred approach of the voluntary day centre meant they adapted to her needs, showing how extra training and support within existing services can act as a catalyst for future development.

Mrs Smith's progressing illness began to manifest itself in problems concerning food, personal hygiene, medication, communication and less insight into her difficulties. Care was adapted accordingly, and attempts were made to introduce Mrs Smith to residential respite care, but the lack of specialist provision made this more difficult. The family remained very involved but the increasing emotional and physical strain on them caused tension between them, and at times between one member and the SW. Thus, more family-centred work, and involvement of colleagues, was necessary to ensure that this did not interfere with Mrs Smith's care or put further strain on the family. Chronic problems concerning eating, weight and agitation resulted in Mrs Smith being admitted briefly to residential care, which again could not manage her needs effectively, before moving to long-term hospital care.

Comment

There was no local residential or nursing home care that could meet Mrs Smith's specific needs. Moving her further afield would have cut her off from important family support. However, Mrs Smith did settle in the continuing care setting, which offered a caring, secure, yet stimulating environment as she became more disabled by her illness. Again, this facility is one that deals predominantly with older people but also has younger people with dementia and has developed some expertise in this area.

Two and a half years earlier Mrs Smith had expressed a wish to remain at home as long as possible but had accepted that she would eventually need care elsewhere. Family and professionals respected her wishes as far as they could. When she did finally need alternative care those involved were able to pass on a clear picture of who she was, what she liked and what she needed in a setting where it was a continuation of care rather than just 'the end of the line'.

Conclusion

This chapter has argued in favour of specialist social workers to work with younger people with dementia and their families. In England, *The Mental Health National Service Framework* and the *National*

Service Framework for Older People advocate specialist services and suggest they be attached to old age psychiatry departments in the absence of an existing established service.

However, where the social worker is based is an important consideration in planning. Adequate support and supervision are essential to prevent isolation and to ensure the best service in challenging and emotionally draining, although rewarding, work. Location is important when advocacy for their client group and raising awareness among colleagues in mainstream services are vital parts of the social work role. The social worker needs to be flexible, but also part of a multidisciplinary team whilst at the same time being supported by social work colleagues. This ensures that client-centred skills are employed most effectively.

References:

Alzheimer's Society (2000) *Younger People with Dementia: A Guide to Service Development and Provision*. London: Alzheimer's Society (UK).

Harvey RJ (1998) *Young Onset Dementia: Epidemiology, Clinical Symptoms, Family Burden, Support and Outcome*. London: Dementia Research Group.

Kitwood T (1997) *Dementia Reconsidered: the Person Comes First*. Buckingham: Open University Press.

NHSAS (NHS Health Advisory Service) (1996) *Mental Health Services: Heading for Better Care*. London: NHSAS.

Quinn C (1996) *The Care Must be There: Improving services for people with young onset dementia and their families*. London: The Dementia Relief Trust.

Ross C (2000) Presentation on working as a social worker in the Royal Borough of Kensington and Chelsea. Paper presented at an Alzheimer's Society Conference on Younger People with Dementia, London, 23 October.

chapter 8

Day care and outreach interventions

Catherine Byrne, Denise Dickson, Catherine Kinsella and Michelle Murray

Day care and outreach services were introduced at the inception of the Carisbrooke service, on a much smaller scale than our present numbers. It was initially envisaged that the need for community outreach would be greater than that for day care. We identified the need through the clients, the majority of whom lived alone. Outreach was tailored to an individual's needs. Staff were able to spend up to three hours with clients individually, helping them maintain social contact within their community and to help them regain and maintain contact with family members and friends. Outreach hours were also used to help with daily living tasks.

Environment

The day care centre is at Carisbrooke in Central Manchester. Its central location in Manchester makes access relatively easy. Entrance is via stairs or lift and there are five small rooms (lounge/TV room, smoking room, snooker room, dining room and kitchen) available for client use. The kitchen is used by some of our clients who are able to make their own refreshments. Because of limited space the rooms have multiple uses. The lounge/TV room is used for the relaxation and exercise groups and group discussions. The dining room doubles as our craft/baking room. Multiple use of these rooms limits the time spent on activities. The smoking room is also used for some art and craft work, although this has its limitations because the atmosphere can be quite unpleasant at times for non-smokers. There is a snooker room, where clients can sometimes find a quiet corner to relax away from the larger groups. The doors of our day care service are not locked. Although there is a security guard at the entrance to the building good levels of supervision of all our day care users are needed so that they do not leave the unit until they are supposed to. This sometimes takes up staff time and limits what can be done, but it is an important consideration when designing a unit, particularly one like Carisbrooke which is not linked to inpatient facilities where security arrangements are more embedded.

Transport

When the Carisbrooke service first began, clients were transported to and from day care by our staff. Although this worked well initially, as our service grew it became increasingly difficult to meet the demand for personal transportation, much of which was done by two members of part-time staff who worked from 9.30 am until 2.30 pm. In practice, clients would arrive at around 11.00 am and have to leave by 1.45 pm in order to be taken home. A minibus was not the answer as our client group is spread across the city, resulting in some clients being subjected to inordinately long journeys. Issues of transport are an important consideration. We now use a taxi firm contracted by the main organization. This has worked well in general, but has not been without its problems. On occasion, clients have been dropped off at the wrong address because the driver has taken instructions from the client rather than follow the written information that he/she has been given. Not all clients can be transported by taxi. Some need to be escorted either in a taxi or a staff vehicle.

Timetable

Our timetable (Table 8.1) is jointly devised by staff and clients and is regularly reviewed. When referrals are accepted to day care an attempt is made to match client needs to the timetable.

Relaxation

The relaxation group is an opportunity for clients to reflect on how they are feeling in a quiet and safe environment. The session begins with a hand or neck and shoulder massage given by a member of staff to each client individually. This is followed by deep breathing exercises and the Laura Mitchell method of muscular relaxation (Mitchell, 1984). This technique is used as it is simple for clients to follow. Relaxing music is played throughout the session, a favourite being Enya and other Celtic music. The session always happens at the same time and follows a similar format so that the clients become familiar with the routine.

Baking

Baking is an excellent activity as it uses familiar skills, stimulates the senses and has a good end-product. We have found that some male

Table 8.1 Carisbrooke day care centre timetable

	Monday	Tuesday	Wednesday	Thursday	Friday
Morning	Exercise	Baking		Allotment Baking	Art and craft work
Afternoon	Reminiscence Discussion	Allotment Quiet activity	Men's group	Relaxation	Outings Current affairs

clients who have not had the opportunity to cook before have really enjoyed this activity and have been pleasantly surprised at their success. Baking can also help to orientate clients to the time of year. We try to identify seasonal ingredients, such as summer fruits for puddings, treacle and apples for autumn events, such as Halloween, spices, etc. for Christmas cakes and puddings. On occasion, we plan with clients to bake cakes to take home for special occasions, such as a family member's birthday.

Art and craft sessions

The opportunity is always available for service users to choose their preferred art and craft activity. However, experience has shown that people prefer and benefit from an organized and structured approach to the sessions. This gives group members a stability that aids short-term memory in various degrees depending on the individual. For most of the group, the Friday art session is now an established part of the week, although a reminder is often required as to the content of the session, especially if the work is progressing over a number of sessions.

In choosing activities, we consider to some extent the abilities of the individual members of the group, although we find that with adequate support most difficulties can be overcome and pleasing results achieved. Although techniques used can appear to be fairly basic and reminiscent of schooldays, the subject matter is always appropriately adult in nature, often geared towards functional and/or decorative items for the unit, or for sale to raise funds.

Whilst formal assessment is not the main function of the group, an individual's progress can be monitored indirectly. For example, short-term memory may be assessed by a person's ability to remember and follow instructions; detailed work of various kinds can highlight someone's visuospatial difficulties and concentration can be assessed by the individual's capacity for 'sticking to the task'. With this in mind, it is vital to have the session planned and fairly short in length, allowing, where possible, for the task to reach a satisfactory finishing point by the end of the session. This gives the participant a structured beginning and end to a task.

The art sessions then are 'designed' to be a time when people with a variety of artistic abilities have the opportunity to work together in a relaxed environment, while staff can monitor function and assess ability informally.

Outings

As shown in Table 8.1, there is a range of activities on offer. Additionally, occasional outings occur. These can be to a:

- local park,
- local market,
- garden centre,
- museum,
- special event, (e.g. street festival), or
- short walk.

Events like these require little formal organization but do depend on factors such as staffing level weather and client requests.

Several larger-scale events also occur through the year, with the aim of bringing all our clients together to enjoy a social event. This is more time consuming and requires great organizational ability. These have included:

- an annual Christmas lunch at a hotel,
- stately home and garden visit,
- the Blackpool illuminations,
- Granada Television studio tour,
- seaside visit,
- a safari park.

These events are quite expensive and are not funded from our budget. They are paid for by donations and fund-raising. Throughout the year we also aim to celebrate religious festivals and events via the centre's activities. Evaluation of our day care service has been undertaken (see Chapter 14). Despite the obvious problems with the environment and the transport system it is apparent that the clients enjoy and value the day care service. A number of attenders have tried other day care centres, but unsuccessfully. Sometimes, this is because younger people may be offered attendance at a centre for older people, which they find inappropriate; in other instances, the skills of the staff in working with younger people with dementia and persistence pay off. Both the centre and personal outreach have contributed in important ways to the quality of life of both client and carer.

Reference

Mitchell L (1984) *Healthy Living over 55*. London: John Murray.

chapter 9

Support for patients

Emma Shlosberg

The effectiveness of providing emotional support in a group format is well recognized (Whitaker, 2001). Until the late 1990s, there had been limited research aimed at understanding the perceptions and experiences of people with dementia. However, more recently, there has been increased interest in the use of psychotherapeutic approaches with people with dementia. Although practices are now moving in the right direction, a major criticism of dementia care has been that it has denied most people with dementia any opportunity to react to or address their condition. In keeping with contemporary expectations of more patient involvement in care this is changing and it is anticipated that sharing the diagnosis with those who have dementia will become the norm.

Public perception of dementia tends to focus on the negative aspects. Although some of these views may be true, it seems that other equally important truths are often overlooked. First and foremost, younger people with dementia are people first and not 'cases' of dementia (Stokes, 2000). Also, they typically maintain good health and functioning for several years.

Without attempting to summarize the wealth of material or repeating other chapters, it may be helpful to identify their central argument as focusing on the importance of 'personhood' and the development of person-centred approaches (Kitwood and Bredin, 1992). Specifically:

- Communicating with people with dementia.
- Focusing on the retention of skills.
- Increasing quality of life.
- Encouraging/supporting relative well-being.
- Attempting to understand the subjective experiences of people with dementia.
- Creating an environment that promotes 'personhood'.

There is increasing clinical and research interest in providing emotional support for people with dementia by drawing on psychotherapeutic and counselling skills. Depression is a common reaction to loss and will be compounded by a chronic and progressive illness such as dementia. There is currently a division in the literature about whether depression in dementia is a result of facing the reality of having dementia or lacking the opportunity to engage in conversation about it. If the latter is true then support groups offer potential benefits.

Historically, support groups have been effective in helping people deal with a range of life transitions. Support groups that combine education and emotional expression are widely available to carers of people with dementia and there is no reason why individuals with dementia do not have 'analogous needs for connection with and affirmation by others' (Yale, 1995).

This chapter is divided into two sections. The first offers some thoughts and practical advice on the issues to consider when starting a support group. The subsequent section describes the alcohol-related dementia support group work carried out in the Carisbrooke (Manchester) service.

Issues to consider when starting a support group

Group work is difficult but can be rewarding for both participants and facilitators alike providing it has been well-planned and thought out.

The following areas, therefore, require particular consideration before embarking.

Venue and arrangement of the room

The difficulty in finding suitable accommodation is acknowledged but, if possible, groups of this nature would benefit from taking place in community environments, away from hospital or other institutional settings. The room should be made as comfortable and informal as possible (e.g. by placing the chairs in an open circle to help facilitate discussion).

Transport

Reliable transport arrangements to and from the group will need to be carefully thought out, and some types of transport may mean that cost implications and careful coordination will need to be considered. Alternatively, caregivers may be in a position to transport care recipients, in which case close liaison with carers will be required.

Group facilitators

There are advantages to deciding who and how many group facilitators there will be initially as this will allow collaborative planning, joint decision-making and will also allow facilitators to gain an understanding of their compatibility.

Co-facilitating shares the group responsibilities and allows one-to-one work within the group to take place if necessary. Also, on a more practical level, it is useful to know that someone else is available to run the group in the event of an emergency.

Group participants

Who is the group for? Will there be separate groups for individuals with different types of dementia or will a more general group for all younger people with dementia work?

Participant selection is extremely important and a key to success. Prior to the group starting, it is important to meet with co-facilitators and make some clear decisions about inclusion and exclusion criteria.

A group membership of six to nine participants is the ideal. Ways and means of advertising and recruiting participants will also require consideration and may require liaison with other health care providers or voluntary agencies.

Having a preliminary one-to-one meeting with possible group participants is often useful not only to ascertain whether that person is suitable to participate, but also as it allows one to prepare prospective participants by explaining the nature of the group. Most participants will have some reservations about entering the group; it is therefore important to allow these to be aired in this meeting prior to the group, allowing any myths or misconceptions to be dealt with. Obviously, any individuals that display extreme anxiety in group situations may need to be excluded. Informed consent to participate can also be gained at this meeting, ideally with written details to supplement verbal accounts. It may also be helpful to discuss the group with primary caregivers and provide them with information about the nature and practicalities of the group.

Group structure

Consideration will need to be given to the group structure. The ethos of support groups for people with dementia is to enhance feelings of empowerment. This will therefore require facilitators to work in a less structured way. However, if facilitators are not used to working in this manner this may prove difficult. It is therefore extremely important that the unstructured format is given a chance to work. If group participants cannot work within the structure (possibly due to extreme distress) then the facilitator may need to make some adaptations.

Support groups of this nature generally involve a closed group membership. If an open membership format is preferred then facilitator style may need to be adapted and awareness that the introduction of new group participants may hinder discussions will need to be acknowledged.

Therapist style

The following therapist qualities are essential:

- empathy,
- patience and a willingness to refocus and repeat certain session contents,
- good communication skills and an ability to simplify language,
- familiarity with mental health issues and up to date information about dementia care,
- familiarity with group work would be advantageous.

The therapist needs to be mindful of the participants' initial anxieties and must avoid the group becoming either too threatening or so safe that no issues of significance occur. Use of acceptance, empathic listening and normalization can help to alleviate the emotional distress (e.g. anger, grief and despair) associated with cognitive impairment.

Taking a positive lead role for at least the first session will probably be necessary, but it is envisaged that as the group develops and becomes more cohesive the need for a leader will diminish and sessions may be less structured. The power and benefits of group work are usually illustrated by the interaction between group members, which may only require a few words of encouragement and support from the facilitators. At other times, the facilitator may need to take a more directive stance. The facilitator will also need a sense of when not to intervene and it may be important not to interrupt too often.

Aims

These will obviously vary depending on the individuals attending the group but broadly include:

- Supporting people in addressing emotional reactions to having dementia.
- Encouraging the sharing and comparison of feelings and experiences of people with dementia.
- Allowing people with dementia to feel that they are being heard.

- Providing an opportunity for people with dementia to express feelings of loss.
- Strengthening the individual's ability to deal with losses.
- Allowing participants to decide on session contents as this enables them to feel more empowered.
- Building up adaptive coping strategies.
- Allowing participants to give and receive constructive feedback.

Session format

If group participants do not feel safe in the group then they will not participate. This may result in a high drop-out rate or alternatively they may find ways to insulate themselves from the experience.

The establishment of group ground rules (known in the therapy world as the 'dynamic administration' of the group) helps to maximize the chances that group participants will feel safe and secure in the group and provides norms which define acceptable and unacceptable ways of behaviour in the group. It is important that the group rules are devised in collaboration with group participants. Not only will this facilitate feelings of empowerment but it will also encourage participants to take an active role early on in the group. It may be helpful to provide written summaries of the ground rules and group boundaries and re-emphasize them at the beginning of each group meeting.

Supervision

Extra time after each group session should be allowed to discuss the group dynamics, such as how participants react to one another and the facilitators, whether any subgroups have developed within the larger group, etc. Although not always available, it would be advantagous if a supervisor who has not been involved in the group could be present after the meeting to provide objectivity. Much can be gained from reviewing a group once it has ended. Questions such as 'what lessons have been learnt?' and 'how could that have been improved?' may facilitate one's own learning and also be of benefit to future groups.

Record-keeping

This may be required by managers and could include brief notes about themes and individual attendance records.

Examples of session contents

- Allow individuals to tell their own story with the prompt: 'When did you first notice you had a memory problem?' It is the facilitator's role to elicit what meanings individuals attach to their problems and how other people react.
- Getting to know each other exercises. Gather ideas from participants ensuring that the activities are age-appropriate and relevant.
- Encourage participants to develop a list of group goals (i.e. what they hope to achieve by the end of the group).

Although the nature of the group encourages participants to take an active role in setting the agenda, it may be helpful for group facilitators to consider and prepare some information on certain discussion topics for the earlier sessions. Some examples include:

- educational material about dementia,
- relaxation exercises,
- information about practical or financial assistance,
- list of useful voluntary organizations/contact names,
- practical ways to assist with memory problems (e.g. external memory aides).

Group evaluation

Administering some form of outcome measure is extremely important but is made difficult by the lack of suitable measures. One needs to remember that although support groups may produce some therapeutic change, this is not one of the primary objectives. Therefore, measurement of anxiety or depression may not be deemed appropriate. With participants' consent, sessions could be tape-recorded, transcribed and subjected to qualitative analysis, although this requires training and is time consuming.

Group facilitators should also keep a logbook. Details of all the group sessions including any handouts that were provided should also be kept for all the issues that were raised in group sessions or in supervision. It is often useful to keep a record of the themes that emerged through the interaction of participants and how participants and/or facilitators contributed to and responded to them.

The next section of this chapter focuses on one of the support groups conducted at the Carisbrooke Younger Persons Dementia Service.

The Carisbrooke alcohol-related dementia support group

Background to the service
Alcohol-related dementia is a common referral received by the Carisbrooke service and may reflect the geographical area, which covers an inner city where poverty is high and as such, problems of poor self-care, poor nutrition and poor attention to health may predominate.

Facilitators
There are three facilitators, a clinical psychologist, an occupational therapist and a support worker.

Venue and transport
The young onset dementia service is based in the community and fortunately has access to a separate large room away from the day care centre. The room is located on the first floor with a lift available. If participants are not already attending for day care, taxis are provided.

Participant selection
Prior to the group starting, the facilitators meet to discuss the recruitment of participants. It was decided to pool participants from those already attending day care, as potential benefits, such as reduced anxiety due to familiar faces and surroundings, were envisaged.

Current day care attendees are discussed in relation to the agreed inclusion criteria:

- diagnosis,
- levels of insight,
- degree of cognitive impairment (based on clinical judgement not screening tools),
- whether there is a willingness to discuss their diagnosis and the associated impact on their life,
- ability to communicate (i.e. able to sustain a conversation, able to express him/herself, able to comprehend others),
- someone who will not feel overly threatened in a group situation.

Based on this information, a number of suitable participants were gathered. Interestingly, participants had diagnoses of either alcohol-related dementia or Alzheimer-type dementia. It was therefore decided to run two streams of support groups dependent on diagnosis. The alcohol-related dementia support group is discussed here. Considering the nature of the group an additional inclusion criteria was established, specifically, a willingness to discuss and acknowledge his/her past or current alcohol dependency.

Facilitators familiar with the clients provided a consent form and also a brief information sheet and consent to contact carers was also gained. The process of participant selection is illustrated in the flow diagram (see Figure 9.1).

Group style

From the outset, it was decided that the group would be collaborative in nature with participants deciding on the style and structure of the group sessions. It was run as a closed group due to the likelihood of sensitive issues being raised. A time-limited format of six sessions was agreed upon with each group meeting lasting for approximately an hour and a half. A short break was provided allowing for smoking or refreshments. If participants were unable to express a preference for discussion topics, facilitators offered some

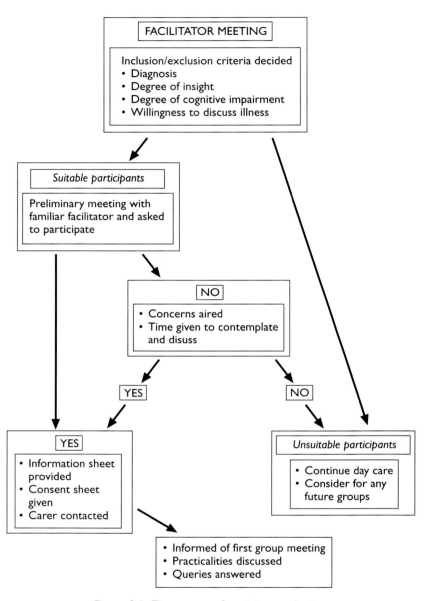

Figure 9.1 *The process of participant selection.*

suggestions. The sample session contents provided by Yale (1995) served as a resource.

Ground rules

Group ground rules were mainly devised by participants and included:

- Keeping information within the group.
- Listening to others.
- Allowing others to talk.
- Being honest.
- Avoiding the use of offensive language.
- Not smoking during the group session.
- Not being under the influence of alcohol whilst attending the group.

Group timetable

Group 1   *Introductions*
          Explanation of meetings
          Getting acquainted
          Ground rules
          General sharing of experiences

Group 2   *Alcohol-related dementia*
          Educational material
          Allowing individuals to 'tell their stories'

Group 3   *Relationship issues*
          Adjusting to changes in our lives
          Coping with other people's reactions
          Family issues

Group 4   *Coping with changes*
          Acknowledging differences
          Sharing coping strategies
          Dealing with stress and anxiety
          Relaxation

Group 5	*Building on positives*
	Building on strengths
	Finding activities → pleasure and mastery
	Maintaining good health
	Improving quality of life
Group 6	*Review and endings*
	Group evaluation
	Expressing feelings about the ending

Attendance/Drop-outs

All group participants attended every session and there were no drop-outs.

However, one participant died during the course of meetings and so additional time was allocated to allow expression of emotions and the expression of grief.

Group evaluation

Questions arose as to what to evaluate. This was not a therapy group so measurement of depression or anxiety was not thought appropriate. The aim of the group was to provide an environment in which individuals felt supported, valued and listened to, but to measure this in a quantitative sense proved difficult due to a lack of appropriate measures. Each participant was therefore asked to evaluate the group with a user-friendly measure designed to assess the content of group sessions; space was available for comments, enabling the collation of qualitative material. This measure was administered at the end of each group meeting. It was also important for group facilitators to evaluate the group with respect to issues that were raised and how they were subsequently dealt with. Armed with both forms of evaluation it is hoped that future groups can be held and modifications made based on the lessons learned.

Lessons learnt

■ Certain group members knew each other well prior to the group starting. Initial anxieties centred around whether the group would function as a whole or whether subgroups would be formed. Fortunately, the group functioned as a cohesive unit but awareness of this possible division would need to be considered for future groups.

■ Having individuals with a diagnosis of alcohol-related dementia allowed for more detailed and specific discussions and enhanced feelings of 'not being alone'.

■ The mix of participants (current levels of alcohol consumption varied between group members) worked well in this group and was supported by qualitative data: 'Coming to these sessions strengthens my resolve not to drink'.

■ Due to time constraints the group was held monthly. It has been decided to run future groups on at least a fortnightly, but preferably weekly, basis as it is envisaged that this will allow for maximum consolidation of any gains made.

■ Feedback from carers would be an interesting avenue to pursue.

■ A time-limited support group is one interesting way to chart the individual's process through the process of dementia.

■ Joint facilitating proved extremely useful not just on a practical basis but also allowed for skill-mixing.

References

Kitwood T, Bredin K (1992) *Person to Person*. Loughton: Gale Centre Publications.

Stokes G (2000) *Challenging Behaviour in Dementia. A Person Centred Approach*. Bicester: Winslow.

Whitaker DS (2001) *Using Groups to Help People*. Brunner Routledge.

Yale R (1995) *Developing Support Groups for Individuals with Early Stage Alzheimer's Disease. Planning, Implementation and Evaluation*. London: Health Professions Press.

chapter 10

Support for carers

Jackie Kindell

There has been a carers group for younger people with dementia for over five years at Carisbrooke, Manchester. The carers attending this group have helped to explain why this is a valuable part of service delivery and their comments are in italics. Following on from this, there is a practical guide to setting up groups of this nature.

It is well documented that carers looking after people with dementia experience high levels of burden. The burden is multifaceted including psychological, financial, physical and social factors (George and Gwyther, 1986):

- *Psychological/emotional.* The stress of caring, can lead to psychiatric symptoms such as anxiety and depression (Livingston, 1996; Harvey, 1998).
- *Financial.* There can be a loss of income from the person with dementia and the carer, and paying for care can be costly.
- *Physical.* Caring can be very tiring, and along with stress, can eventually lead to physical health problems (Bergman Evans, 1994).
- *Social.* There is decreased opportunity for the carer to engage in society and often a reduction in contact with both family and friends (Wenger, 1994).

For these reasons, services need to be built around not just the needs of the person with dementia, but also the family.

Why are support groups helpful?

Carers need a network of support and information, and carers support groups are part of this. At the Carisbrooke Younger Persons Dementia Service, we felt that the carers group was not an alternative to one-to-one support, counselling and information, but a complement to this, and tapped into the caring experience in a different way.

Not all carers want to attend the support group, but some find regular meetings with other younger carers a very supportive experience. Some of them also attend other support groups for carers of people with dementia of all ages, reporting that these are also helpful. However, others have found them either very distressing, or just not able to meet their needs. All those who attend the group feel that only other carers of younger people could truly understand their experience, for example: *'You've got to live with it to understand it'* and *'Nobody [at the group] is judging you, or thinking what a stupid thing to say . . . because they're experiencing it'*. For this reason, carers attend the group from a wide area because of the lack of such groups in their locality. We feel it is a success of the group that people are willing to travel such distances.

Over the years, group members have become extremely supportive of each other. They have been able to express a range of emotions, such as sadness, fear, guilt and anger, which other carers can relate to, in an open and non-judgemental setting, e.g. *'If you feel guilty about thinking something . . . you say it here and someone says 'I've thought that too'. . . it really helps'*. Releasing emotions that are often bottled up helps, e.g.: *'It helps you get it off your chest', 'Once you've said it . . . it doesn't feel so bad',* and *'these meetings help put it in perspective'*. At times, the opportunity to laugh about recent predicaments together, is a powerful way to cope, e.g. *'You can cry with each other, laugh with each other . . . and it is exactly what it says . . . support'*.

Carers are often able to advise and help each other, and this, in some instances, is more helpful than professional advice; perhaps it has more credibility for some carers, e.g. *'We help each other perhaps get round problems or give each other information'*. Admitting and hearing that no one was the perfect 'textbook' carer was important, e.g. *'To meet other carers is a great support, to find that other people get just as tired or just as impatient or whatever'*. Sharing ideas about caring and services is particularly important in young onset dementia, where people often receive a low level of services (Baldwin, 1994a), and the care package is a patchwork of services from health, social services, voluntary and private agencies. Carers often first hear about services from each other and they can show each other 'around the system', helping both access and acceptance of services. Carers of younger people with dementia can be uncomplaining, or feel guilty about accepting services, often caring with little help, in very difficult circumstances (Baldwin, 1994b). At the group, carers help each other with this. For example, the issue of respite care is often raised, along with the guilt associated with accepting it. Carers advise each other that accepting respite is not due to failure on their part, and explain the practical ways in which it can help the situation.

Professionals should be aware that there is often a worry that support groups may concentrate on the negative side of caring. However, many of our carers are keen to keep themselves and others positive, e.g. *'I'm sort of at the beginning stage and it's reassuring that they've come through this and we're all there . . .'*.

The group strongly believes that being a carer of a younger person with dementia brings its own particular set of burdens and challenges. Issues that frequently arise in the group and provoke discussion include:

■ *The unexpected nature of the diagnosis*
  Many carers comment on the shock at a diagnosis that both they and others, including professionals, associate with old age, e.g. *'The doctor came to visit my husband and when I answered the door he said 'are you the daughter?', I had to explain he was my husband, he'd obviously not read the notes and noticed his age . . . I was so upset'*. At times, carers comment on the resentment they feel about the illness, e.g. *'It's not right . . . we're in the middle of life, it's not fair'*.

■ *The diagnostic process*

For some, the diagnostic process may have been long and drawn out, because dementia is not expected in younger people, e.g. *'He [the doctor] kept saying it was 'the change of life', but it just didn't make sense, she had more problems than that, but I couldn't get him to take it seriously'*. Others comment that they found it difficult to get precise information, e.g. *'You ask questions but you just get blank stares, or they talk around it, you just want a definite answer'*.

■ *Giving up work*

Because of the dementia, the person had to give up work, losing his/her income, often at a time they would have been accruing significant funds for their pension, thus putting a financial burden on the family, both now, and for the future. With the burden of caring the spouse/carer may then also have to give up work. Some carers report that employers were very helpful, e.g. *'The supermarket was so good, they used to pick him up each day and then bring him home, they kept him on longer really than they had to'*. Whereas others report the opposite, e.g. *'I couldn't believe he'd worked so hard all those years . . . and they treated him like that'*, and *'If she'd only been a bit more flexible I could have carried on working and looked after him'*.

■ *Telling the children*

For those with young children, carers have to explain and support them in understanding, and coming to terms with the diagnosis, e.g. *'I feel so sorry, she's only ten and he shouts at her if she picks up the letters off the mat, he's like a child . . . She's losing her dad, but what can I do?'*

■ *Isolation*

Carers may find themselves isolated at a time in life they expected to be still active in the workplace and in their social life. Whilst some report that friends have been a tower of strength, others report that friends do not understand or slowly withdraw, e.g. *'He used to do everything for everybody . . . but now they don't want to know and it hurts so much'*, and *'You certainly find out who your real friends are'*. Some do not want to burden friends with talking about the situation—*'because they can't cope with our upset'*. The relationship with the person who has dementia changes, and carers often miss the companionship, along with a lack of appreciation of the tasks that they do. Others comment on the changes to the sexual, intimate side of the relationship, e.g. *'I miss the sex of course . . . but I really just wish he'd turn round and give me a hug'*.

■ *Dealing with challenging behaviour*
The person with dementia may be fit, healthy and strong, but display challenging behaviours that can be hard to deal with, e.g. *'because he's so fit if he gets out he can walk for miles . . . and of course no one in the street would suspect there was anything wrong with him'*, and *'He's so strong . . . and big . . . I used to get really frightened when he got angry'*. Psychological and behavioural symptoms were common in Harvey's (1998) study of young onset dementia, and this has been particularly associated with caregiver stress (Donaldson et al, 1997).

■ *Lack of specialist services*
The lack of appropriate services for younger people with dementia often means either attending units for younger people with mental illness, or centres for the elderly, and this can bring home the sadness of the situation, e.g. *'She was sat there in the middle of all these old people . . . I don't think she noticed but I found it heartbreaking'*.

■ *The present and the future*
Carers know that the young person with dementia will eventually die from the illness, and that they are likely to have a large slice of life ahead of them after this. This brings a range of emotions, including 'making memories' while it is possible but also ensuring life goes on, e.g. *'OK we've read the books . . . we've got the information but we've got to get on with our lives still . . . now's the time to make memories'* and *'I'm determined not to be a victim of this . . . to get through it all . . . and still keep some of me'*.

As professionals, we learn a lot about the effects of caring from the group and we feel this makes us better practitioners. For example, we learnt that when we gave advice it could be taken as criticism of carers, and that sometimes too much advice and information can make an already stressful situation seem more of a burden. Whilst advice and information is important, in some instances, there is no solution or 'caring technique' that can solve the problem at hand, and that what people often need is the space to air feelings.

Practical issues

There are a number of practical issues in setting up a group that are important. These are discussed below.

Time
Following consultation with carers, our group has always been held in the afternoon. However, as some carers may still work, consider whether an evening group would be more appropriate. No time is going to suit everybody, but it is best to ask the carers concerned. We plan for a group of two hours (i.e. 1 pm–3 pm), and staff involved allocate time for setting up, and always allow an hour afterwards to talk to individual carers and tidy up. Equally, one needs to ask carers how often they would like to meet. It may be easy to remember if the group is on the same day, such as the last Tuesday of the month. Our carers opted to meet every six weeks.

Leaving the person with dementia
In order to attend the group many carers have to make arrangements for someone to sit with the person with dementia, or for them to attend day care that day. We are able to help carers with this task by suggesting appropriate services, or directly negotiating with services ourselves. It is important to stress to services that attendance at the group is an essential part of the care package.

Venue
This has been discussed in relation to patient/client groups (Chapter

9). A room with access to tea- and coffee-making facilities is required. It should be private to maintain confidentiality and reduce interruptions, and be comfortable to give an appropriate informal feel. Consider if there is another smaller private room you could take carers to if they are upset or need to talk on an individual basis, if this is a practical possibility. Access to the venue in terms of road, rail and bus routes is important to us because of the distances many carers travel. Adequate and safe parking for vehicles is also important, along with safety at night-time meetings.

Staffing

It is important to have the same staff running the group as carers are able to get to know and trust them. This helps in remembering their stories and they do not have to keep repeating the same information to new people. Consideration should be given as to whether observers, or students, can attend the group. In our situation, we do not allow 'one-off' observers, but do allow students who are on placement at the centre to attend if they can commit to a number of sessions. We usually have three members of staff, and run the group with not less than two, so we can meet and greet people, introduce and support new members, help make and serve drinks, look after speakers and support people on a one-to-one basis, if they get upset. Careful consideration should be given to whether the group is going to be run by professional staff, or by carers, or volunteers. At times in our group, emotions run high, and we feel that professional input is vital to facilitate, step in and direct when needed, and ensure information given is accurate. We are also able to identify those carers who are under particular strain and seek advice, counselling or services for them. Following the group, telephone calls are often made to other agencies to make referrals or access information on the carer's behalf. The group is run by a nurse, speech and language therapist and an occupational therapist and this helps provide a range of specialist skills and advice. All have experience of working with dementia and of running groups.

The name of the group

Consider if the group should be called a 'relatives group' or a 'carers group' or named after the service. Should it include the term 'dementia'? If the diagnosis has not yet been confirmed, consider whether it is appropriate for carers to attend at this stage or perhaps later. As our service was for people after diagnosis, we are able to call our group the 'Carisbrooke Younger Persons Dementia Carers Group'.

Criteria for attendance

'Caring for someone with a diagnosis of dementia who is under 65 years' is our criterion. We accept carers from areas that our service does not cover, if they are willing to travel. Carers can refer themselves or others can make contact on their behalf, and then we would contact the carer. If the person with dementia then reaches his/her 65th birthday, attendance at the group can still continue, even though currently, the person with dementia him/herself may be transferred to older people's services. If the person with dementia dies the carer can also continue to attend. In both instances, we have left the decision up to the carer concerned, and this has worked out well. However, when groups have been running for a long time, it may be necessary to consider if this is appropriate, as for example, having a significant number of ex-carers changes the dynamics of the group. Supporting carers to develop their own lives after the death of the person with dementia, however, is seen as an important part of the service and the group.

Numbers

Our group usually runs with six to ten carers. The numbers vary above and below this on occasions, but we feel that it is important not to fall below four carers to keep the group viable.

Publicity

We produced a leaflet describing the group containing contact information and a map, and sent it to various agencies including Social Services, the local Alzheimer's Society, the Memory Clinic, Old

Age Psychiatry, Psychiatry for Working Age Adults, and the Neurology department. Links were made with various agencies at a national level including the Alzheimer's Society and the Pick's Disease Support Group. By doing this, we hope that carers can hear about our service from a variety of sources. We also have a carers mailing list and send a reminder two weeks before each group outlining the topic and date.

Introduction to the group

As discussed above we have an open referral system and people hear about the group from a range of sources. Some carers are quite happy to come along themselves the first time, after making an initial telephone contact. Others are less confident, and so we arrange for a member of staff to either meet them, or bring them to the group. Occasionally, we visit people at home, prior to the group, to discuss the group's aims, etc. to encourage attendance.

Format

The group begins with having a cup of tea or coffee and an informal chat as people arrive. Following this, there is either a speaker, or a discussion around a given theme, usually for about an hour or so, finishing with another drink and time to talk. We quickly found that the informal conversations were as important as the speaker, and some groups we designate as 'catching up' or 'socials' to allow this to occur. At times, it is hard to stop discussions once they are under way, and staff have to be assertive or use skilled humour, to ensure quiet for the speaker to begin!

Aim of the group

Consider if the group is aiming to give information and advice, or is aiming more to share feelings and experiences, or both. At the outset we felt that both were important, but initially concentrated on the former until the group had got to know each other, and were comfortable enough to talk openly. As carers became more familiar with the group, we were able to move from formal presentations to more discussion around a particular theme. At some point, ownership of the group seemed to pass to the carers, and the informal emotional support provided from carer to carer became the most powerful and valuable resource. In addition, the carers became able to plan the information or topic they wanted to talk about.

Ground rules

Again, this has been covered in the previous chapter (Chapter 9) in relation to patient/client groups. Suggested rules for a carers group include:

- Confidentiality.
- There's no such thing as a stupid question.
- Respect for everyone's views.

It may be useful to have these on a chart or laminated card on the wall in the room, to refer to. At times it can be hard to get people to stick to the topic at hand, for example, asking speakers questions they cannot answer, or bringing up topics not relevant to the discussion. In such instances, it may be useful to have a large piece of paper for writing 'future topics/questions', to indicate they cannot be dealt with now, but can be addressed in future meetings.

Other functions of the group

Over the years, the group has been a useful and powerful place to access carers' views regarding services. Many managers have found the group useful and humbling, with respect to the carers' knowledge and ability to convey their feelings. It is, however, worth remembering that 'consultation fatigue' may set in when carers are asked about services again and again, but no feedback is given, or worse still, services do not change as a result. It was because of the lack of services for this group that some of our carers formed a smaller action group to lobby for better services, for example, writing letters to managers in health and social services, and politicians at local and national levels. This group fed back to the carers group, although it was important to keep the two groups separate as they had different functions.

Suggestions for topics

Some of the topics which have been covered in past years, and the speakers we have used are shown in Tables 10.1 and 10.2.

It is hard to measure the clinical effectiveness of carers groups, although they are often favoured by services. A small qualitative study of carers attending our service reported positively about it (Chapter 14). Certainly, to ensure such groups are effective they need to meet regularly, and be of the highest quality (Gilhooly, 1984).

Table 10.1

Discussion topics
- To tell or not to tell (the person their diagnosis)
- Why is caring stressful?
- Why do I sometimes feel guilty?
- How do you tell the children?
- How do you tell people about the diagnosis?
- What helps me to relax?
- What services do you find helpful?
- What does 'a carer' mean—Are you 'a carer'?
- What is the one thing I will do for *myself* this year?

Table 10.2 Topics for speakers

Topic	Speaker
What is dementia?	Psychiatrist/Specialist nurse
The different types of dementia	Psychiatrist/Specialist nurse
Specific drug treatments for dementia	Psychiatrist/Specialist nurse
Other drugs used in psychiatry (e.g. antidepressants, antipsychotics, etc.)	Psychiatrist/Specialist nurse
Welfare benefits advice	Welfare rights officer
The role of Social Services	Social worker
Respite care	Social worker/Nurse
Roles of professionals (e.g. nurse, occupational therapist, physiotherapist or speech and language therapist, psychologist, social worker, etc.)	Relevant discipline
Psychological treatments in dementia	Psychologist
Management of challenging behaviour	Psychologist/Nurse
Communication problems	Speech and language therapist
Activities	Occupational therapist
Stress management techniques	Occupational therapist/Nurse
Legal issues	Solicitor/Local Alzheimer's Society
Safety in the home	Occupational therapist
Nutrition	Dietitian
Moving and handling	Physiotherapist
Keeping fit and active	Physiotherapist
Patient's rights and the Mental Health Act	Approved social worker
Meal-time difficulties	Speech and language therapist/Occupational therapist
Alternative medicine	Aromatherapist/Holistic therapist
Voluntary agencies (e.g. Crossroads)	Relevant agency
Holidays for people with dementia	Alzheimer's Society

References

Baldwin RC (1994a) Service experiences of people with presenile dementia. *Int J Geriat Psychiatry* **9:** 507.

Baldwin RC (1994b) Acquired cognitive impairment in the presenium. *Psychiat Bull* **18:** 463–465.

Bergman Evans B (1994) A health profile of spousal Alzheimer's caregivers: depression and physical health characteristics. *J Psychosocial Nurs Mental Health Services* **32:** 25–30.

Donaldson C, Tarrier N, Burns A (1997) The impact of the symptoms of dementia on caregivers. *Br J Psychiatry* **170:** 62–68.

George LK, Gwyther LP (1986) Caregiver well-being: a multidimensional examination of family caregivers of demented adults. *Gerontologist* **3:** 253–259.

Gilhooly MLM (1984) The social dimensions of senile dementia. In Hanley I, Hodge J (eds) *Psychological Approaches to Care of the Elderly.* London: Croom Helm.

Harvey RJ (1998) Young Onset Dementia: epidemiology, clinical symptoms, family burden, support and outcome. Dementia Research Group. (http://dementia.ion.ucl.ac.uk/).

Livingston G, Manela M, Katana C (1996) Depression and other psychiatric morbidity in carers of elderly people living at home. *Br Med J* **312:** 153–156.

Wenger GC (1994) Support networks and dementia. *Int J Geriat Psychiatry* **9:** 181–194.

chapter 11

Support for families

Kenneth Garrod

In 1984, a group of people from several different disciplines working within the Old Age Psychiatry Service in Central Manchester established a clinic that offered a family therapy service to older people with mental health problems and their families. Over the years of its operation the Central Manchester Family Therapy Team (at Carisbrooke) developed substantial knowledge and experience in working with this particular group of people, almost half of whom had a diagnosis of a dementing illness. The work of the team with the families of older people with dementia has been described elsewhere (Benbow et al, 1993). The creation of the Younger Persons Dementia Service within the larger service five years ago, coupled with the development nurse (Michelle Murray) becoming a member of the family team, led to the conclusion that some of the younger users and their families might also benefit from the particular kind of intervention the team offered. Although thus far the family team has only worked with a relatively small number of families who have a younger member with dementia, its intervention has already shown itself to be of benefit and it is planned that this new aspect of the team's work will continue. This chapter will describe the general approach of the family team to family therapy and indicate the nature of family work it has already carried out with older people with mental health problems and younger individuals with dementia. It will briefly describe the operation of its clinic and will illustrate that work with a case example of one of the families referred from the Younger Persons Dementia Service.

The approach of the Central Manchester (Carisbrooke) Family Therapy Team

Family therapy emerged during the latter half of the last century as an effective way of helping people and their families with a variety of problems. It came to be seen as an approach that, at the very least, complemented others that focused mainly on interventions with and for the individual. It recognized that people were usually part of a family and that social systems could influence their ability to cope with and adapt to their difficulties, sometimes adversely. Marriott (2000) has described this approach. Family and systems therapy involves working with families and systems of relationships between individuals as the main focus for change and development rather than taking an individual perspective that focuses on the individual *per se.*

Historically, family therapy was a therapeutic approach that initially focused on work with younger families with children and adolescent members and then with the families of younger adults with mental health problems. Along with many other therapies it seemed to view old age as a sterile period when growth, change and development for individuals and their families were severely restricted. As this limited and pessimistic view gradually became replaced by one more positive and less ageist, the possibilities of family therapy with older people began to be explored.

This was the view upon which the inception of the Manchester family team was based. It was a way of recognizing the importance of the family and other relationships in later life in both precipitating difficulties for family members and in allowing changes and growth to occur. It was felt that some patients of the Old Age Psychiatry Service could be most fully assisted if this aspect of their situation were recognized and addressed. Sometimes, despite the best efforts of the various professionals who comprised the multidisciplinary Old Age

Psychiatry team, with the range of interventions and services at their disposal, along with the efforts of the family and carers, insufficient progress was made in helping a patient cope with his/her situation. In these cases, it was often evident that a patient's particular family circumstances were a major inhibiting factor. It was found that family therapy can help some individuals and their families adjust to adverse circumstances. Family therapy would then be indicated when it was felt that a change in the way a family functioned could produce beneficial changes for its members. It is not an intervention that has been used in most cases but it has had a place in the repertoire of the Old Age Psychiatry Service as it is relevant to some individuals and families whose problems had seemed impervious to other interventions.

The families who have used the service

The families who have attended the weekly family therapy clinic have been many and varied and have faced a range of challenges and problems. To give a full description here of their scope and diversity would be impossible. However, the following gives some idea of the kind of work undertaken in the clinic and the kinds of issues that have been addressed by the families who have attended. They have included families that have been struggling with:

- Major events that occur in the history of families such as additions to the family i.e. children or partners, separation and divorce, the departure of key family members, family conflict, bereavement, redundancy, retirement and the onset of physical illness.
- The question of future care provision for an individual family member which can take the form of either the provision of support services in the community or the decision to be cared for in some form of residential accommodation.
- Abuse and neglect in its various forms.
- The mental health of another member of the family apart from the identified patient.

■ The mental health of the identified patient, often someone with a diagnosis of dementia.

The Manchester family team in its work with older people with mental health problems therefore had substantial experience working with many families with a varied range of problems, not least the challenges presented by a family member developing a dementing condition. In the work of its clinic, the team had also developed a set of family therapy procedures, techniques and skills that families in difficulty could benefit from. It seemed a logical progression then to make its services available to the users of the newly formed Younger Persons Dementia Service and their families who might benefit from its service. At the time of writing, five families with a member using the younger persons service have been referred to and been seen by the family team. As this step was taken the team acknowledged that although much of their past experience would be relevant such families could bring with them new challenges and areas of hitherto unencountered difficulties.

It is clear that younger people with dementia and their families will encounter challenges and difficulties different in degree and kind to those outlined above for older people, not least because they will be at an earlier stage in their history. As has been highlighted, younger people are more likely to have partners still living, children at an earlier stage in their development and possibly still dependent. There are different implications for the employment and financial situation of these families. Younger individuals and their families will have a wholly different range of expectations and hopes for the course of their lives than their older counterparts. They are, perhaps, less prepared for what is a progressive and profoundly disabling condition to enter and impact on their families. To quote Cox (1991): 'While it may be possible eventually to accept the reality of dementia in old age, it is often more difficult to accept in the midst of life'.

However, they will also face many of the issues presented by the families of older people albeit in different shapes and forms and with different ramifications for their family life. It was felt by the team that our experience of working with older people on these issues and the way of working we had developed could be of benefit to some of the families whose relatives had become patients of the younger persons service.

The operation of the Family Therapy Clinic

The membership of the Manchester family team has varied over its lifetime but it has always managed to maintain a broad multidisciplinary base. Within its ranks it has included an old age psychiatrist, junior psychiatrists, psychologists, hospital and community-based nurses and social workers. The multidisciplinary nature of the team's membership has been an essential feature of its operation. We have recognized that people from different disciplines, with different personalities, will bring contrasting perspectives to bear on family situations, which can lead to an enrichment of the approaches we offer to families. The team has managed to maintain a core membership of six that meets each week on a Friday morning, usually working with two families during a morning session. This has required considerable commitment on the part of the team members themselves, but the valued support of the service as a whole has continued to recognize the contribution family therapy can make to some of its users and their families.

Most families are seen at Carisbrooke which as well as being the base for the Younger Persons Dementia Service is also the community base of the Old Age Psychiatry Service. Technical facilities, such as a video link, are available at Carisbrooke. In some situations, however, it may be more appropriate to meet with the family in their own home and the team's methods of working can be adapted to this context, although this not usual. Each identified family member is invited to attend and also invited to bring with them anyone who is involved in the situation and can make a contribution. It can be seen from this that our definition of membership of the relevant family system is a wide one and family meetings have included important non-family members such as neighbours, home care workers, nurses and social workers. The number of people who attend a session can vary greatly—ranging from one famous occasion when fourteen family members arrived to working with small family groups, with the identified patient and one other to people on their own! Very often we feel that assembling all the relevant people involved in a family system in one location can have a therapeutic effect of itself.

For different family sessions team members take on different roles. They can either be one of the two co-therapists who work directly with the family, the peer consultant who is responsible for supervising the general conduct of the session, or part of the back-up team who view proceedings by way of a video link and can communicate comments and suggestions directly to the therapists by telephone. It has been suggested that families would find what is a somewhat elaborate formula underpinned with its technological trappings daunting, but our experience is they swiftly acclimatize and engage in the proceedings in an open and generous fashion. The number of times a family attends can vary from a single session to many more spaced over a considerable period of time.

The schools and techniques involved in family therapy are many and varied and the Manchester family team have had the opportunity to evolve what could be described as an eclectic approach to its work. However, a significant influence has been the work of the Milan group, along with the ideas of Tom Anderson concerning reflecting teams. These have been comprehensively described by one of our senior family therapists (Marriott, 2000), based on the work of the team. Descriptions can be found of some of the techniques that the team have found most effective including the use of geneograms, circular questioning, hypothesizing and the use of reflecting teams. Suffice it to say in this context, without going into a detailed description of each individual technique, that they all have the effect of enabling families to develop a range of different perspectives on a situation. It is hoped that this will enable them as individuals and collectively as a family to move to a new and more positive position.

The following case example is based on a case referred to the Manchester family team from the Younger Persons Dementia Service. It illustrates how a family therapy approach can be of assistance to individuals with young onset dementia and their families.

Case study

Mrs A was a woman who developed Alzheimer's disease in her mid-50s and consequently became a patient of the Younger Persons Dementia Service. She and her family were referred to the family team following an incident when it was alleged that she had brandished a knife at one of her grandchildren whilst at her daughter's home. Her action was seen as perhaps being indicative of the underlying conflicts and tensions that existed in her family that were primarily concerned with how the family could best care for and support her.

Mrs A had lost her husband about five years previously. He too had dementia and had been cared for by his family until he died. Mr and Mrs A had three daughters and a son and several grandchildren. The family session was attended by Mrs A, her three daughters, her son and a grandaughter. Shortly after the commencement of the session Mrs A left the room of her own accord and remained in the adjoining premises of the younger persons service. After exploring something of the structure and history of the family there began a discussion of the difficulties they were experiencing particularly in relation to Mrs A's care. It soon became apparent that there were major differences between two of the daughters as to how caregiving was divided between them. This had led to a complete breakdown of communication between different parts of the family and individual family members. The family were given the opportunity to express some of these differences and give vent to some of their distress. It was recognized that this distress in its turn produced a living environment of hostility for Mrs A and a profound disruption in the structure of her care.

In an atmosphere of some considerable distress and hostility the family were encouraged to explore how they had cared for Mr A before he died. Some individuals expressed discomfort that they were revealing difficult family matters to non-family members. This led to further discussion around the basic values they all shared as a family and in particular their desire to prevent Mrs A needing to be admitted to residential care. After a very difficult session the family resolved to re-establish communication with each other and work together to find solutions to their problems and conflicts.

The family only attended the clinic on one occasion. Mrs A remained a patient of the Younger Persons Dementia Service. Family relations and communication improved considerably with the net result that they were able to continue caring for her at home. Attendance at the family clinic had an impact on the family system that contributed to the quality of life experienced by the individual patient.

References

Benbow SM, Marriott A, Morley M et al (1993) Family therapy and dementia; review and clinical experience. *Int J Geriatr Psychiatry* **8:** 717–725.

Cox SM (1991) *Planning Report 1: Pre-senile Dementia: an issue paper for service planners and providers.* Stirling: Dementia Services Development Centre, University of Stirling.

Marriott A (2000) *Family Therapy with Older Adults and their Families.* Bicester, Oxon, UK: Speechmark Publications.

chapter 12

Links with other health services

Sean Page and Robert Baldwin

In this chapter we describe three local health services that are relevant to the operation of a service for younger people with dementia. The first, described by Sean Page, is the Memory Clinic, a resource previously only available in a few teaching centres but now seen increasingly as part of the strategic development of local services for dementia. The second has been discussed in Chapter 2, and is the Cerebral Function Unit and the third the local Old Age Psychiatry Service. Both of these are described by Robert Baldwin.

The Memory Clinic (Sean Page)

Memory clinic models

Services that we would nowadays recognize as memory clinics are relatively new to the UK, having been in existence in small numbers (Wright and Lindesay, 1995) for only the past two decades. They have only recently gained formal recognition as a valuable part of specialist mental health services (DoH, 2001). Originating in the US as a neutral assessment alternative for people with very mild memory impairments, they were aimed at those who felt stigmatized by attending the existing dementia or psychiatric services. The existence of memory clinics is particularly relevant to younger people with a suspected dementia and it is therefore important to have a good working knowledge of them and to develop strong links with them. For example, in Manchester the author (SCP) is on the steering groups of both services.

Memory clinics are a direct response to concerns that clinicians have never taken seriously subjective memory loss in younger people. By doing so the original aim of a memory clinic, to find cases of organic cognitive impairment at as early a stage as possible, has stood the test of time.

Quite quickly, memory clinics became rooted in two specific models. The first is the research-driven memory clinic with a scientific emphasis upon gaining a better understanding of the underlying processes that bring about the onset of a dementia, and developing potentially effective treatments. These clinics strive to identify dementia early on. Those who attend are frequently suitable individuals for emerging therapies and will often be offered an opportunity to take part in clinical trials.

The second model is more service-driven. This is often fuelled by the frustrations of those younger and/or mildly affected people who have had difficulties in gaining access to diagnostic facilities (Luscombe et al, 1998). By pursuing a holistic aim such clinics promote social and psychological research, ultimately helping to bring about the social model of dementia care. Here, the emphasis is upon understanding the experience of people with dementia and their families (Gilleard and Keady, 1998). In so doing, more meaningful dialogue occurs leading to better identification of need. People with dementia are therefore regarded as active participants who should be involved not only in decisions about their care but also about the kind of services that should be provided.

Recently, a third model of memory clinic has arisen as a direct consequence of the licensing of the cholinesterase inhibitor (ChEIs) therapies for Alzheimer's disease. These clinics are charged with taking the ChEIs out of the research arena and managing their introduction into routine clinical practice. As such, the emphasis is upon assessing suitability for treatment, monitoring compliance, tolerance and efficacy, and advising on the discontinuation of treatment.

It is a contentious issue as to whether the treatment-driven clinic may actually warrant the title of 'a memory clinic'. The memory clinic, research- or service-driven, begins with an individual's *subjective* complaint of a memory impairment, which is then assessed within a diagnosis framework. This contrasts with the treatment clinic that begins with the *objective* diagnosis of Alzheimer's disease and is concerned with post-diagnostic intervention.

As well as diagnosing dementia, memory clinics invariably make a variety of other diagnoses of cognitive impairment and also, importantly, of non-dementias that simulate or cause reversible cognitive impairment such as depressive disorder.

The memory clinic process

The composition of the memory clinic team traditionally reflects its assessment and diagnostic activity. More recently, there has been an increased interest in the provision of interventions derived from a more social model of dementia care. Most published accounts suggest that there is a minimum requirement for a physician, usually a psychiatrist, neurologist or geriatrician, to work alongside a specialist nurse or psychologist, with other professionals (occupational therapist, speech therapist, etc.) being brought in as required (Hassiotis and Walker, 2001).

Dependent upon the individual clinic protocol and resources, the process may be community-focused or hospital-based and it may be carried out as a one-stop service or over a number of visits. Despite minor differences in operational methods most memory clinics would follow a similar pattern allowing them to gather sufficient information to make a definitive diagnosis. Essential to each memory clinic would be:

- The taking of a detailed psychiatric and medical history, assessment and evaluation.
- The performing of a physical investigation including blood tests and neuroimaging.
- The delivery of a detailed neuropsychological battery of tests.

■ Consultation to provide feedback on the results obtained and to share the diagnosis.

The memory clinic and national reports

The past two years in England has seen the arrival of National Service Frameworks (NSFs) and they are integral parts of the modernization programme for the National Health Service. The underlying principle of NSFs is to view people as individuals entitled by right to services that are directly related to their needs.

The external reference group for the Mental Health NSF (DoH, 1999), as part of its consensus on the fundamental values that guide service development, stated that specialist services should not only seek to meaningfully involve users and carers, but should be open to learning from this. The NSF for Older People (DoH, 2001) has perhaps identified some of the barriers to this in the past, describing some services as being unresponsive, insensitive or in worst cases, discriminatory.

The NSF for Older People identifies the circumstances in which a specialist service may be required, namely:

■ Where the diagnosis is uncertain.
■ Where a difficult dual diagnosis is being considered, for example, dementia in a person with a learning disability.
■ Where the use of a ChEI is being considered.
■ Where a specialist opinion is required in cases of perhaps testamentary capacity or fitness to drive.

Importantly, the NSF for Older People endorses that services for younger people with dementia should come within its remit, with old age psychiatry services taking a lead.

The NHS Plan (DoH, 1998), as well as introducing a series of NSFs, also created the National Institute for Clinical Excellence (NICE). NICE has the status of a Special Health Authority and a remit to provide guidance for clinicians and patients in relation to new medicines, medical equipment, diagnostic tests and clinical procedures.

One of NICE's recent reports, which has a direct bearing on the memory clinic, concerns guidance on the use of the ChEIs (NICE, 2001). Essentially, before treatment with a ChEI may be initiated the diagnosis of Alzheimer's disease has to be made, in a specialist clinic, following assessment and investigation and based upon standardized diagnostic criteria.

Functions of the memory clinic

Whilst identifying early cases of dementia is the dominant function it is by no means the only one; other functions can be identified:

- *Reassure the 'worried well'*. The trigger for referral is a subjective report of memory impairment. Often, reassurance from a specialist that there is no objective impairment is sufficient intervention although sometimes treatment may be required for underlying anxiety states.
- *Identify reversible causes of dementia or pseudodementia*. The commonest conditions looked for would include hypothyroidism, inadequate vitamin B_{12} levels or depression. This potential to find a reversible cause provides the rationale for medical examination and routine blood sampling being an early part of the memory clinic assessment process.
- *Identify causes of cognitive impairment not caused by a dementia*. Most commonly, this includes non-progressive cases of mild cognitive impairment (MCI), age-associated memory impairment (AAMI) or static conditions related to conditions such as cerebrovascular disease or insults. MCI is identified under the ICD-10 criteria (WHO, 1992) as an objectively identified decline in cognitive performance, the symptoms of which are insufficient to make a diagnosis of a dementia or a delirium. AAMI is defined (Crook et al, 1986) as being a diagnostic term applied to medically, neurologically and psychologically healthy persons, over the age of 50 years, who have experienced a gradual decline in daily tasks that are dependent upon memory.

■ *Effective diagnosis leads to appropriate interventions.* These include introducing pharmacological treatments such as ChEIs and anti-depressants. Providing psychosocial interventions, such as cognitive behaviour therapy or memory training alongside novel therapeutic approaches, is part of this too.

■ *Provide support and advice programmes to those affected by a cognitive impairment.* Traditionally, this has included offering education and support programmes to carers of people with dementia who experience caregiver burden (Donaldson and Burns, 1999). More recently, the emerging social model of dementia care has emphasized the needs of the person with dementia, particularly early dementia, to be included in programmes of support and education (Winning, 1998).

■ *Training and educating others.* Memory clinics are clearly specialist services carrying out a variety of specialist functions. They are repositories of specialist skills, knowledge and experience, and they are at the forefront of developing new medical treatments and increasing the medical understanding of the dementias. Taking all of these factors into account, the memory clinic team has an obligation to make their resources as accessible as possible and to provide training and education.

Accessing the memory clinic

Memory clinics are relatively new to the health service in the UK. The only major survey thus far (Wright and Lindesay, 1995) found only twenty in operation around the country. Although this number has undoubtedly increased with the development of the treatment-driven clinics and political encouragement for early diagnosis, there are no new data currently available.

Access to the memory clinic is therefore initially an issue of geography. The existing clinics are generally associated with the university teaching hospitals in the major cities and people in other areas should be prepared to travel some distance to access this specialist service.

Making a referral to a memory clinic is determined by local protocol. The majority of clinics would require agreement of the patient's primary care physician, although regrettably not all see the value of early diagnosis. Other clinics will accept self-referrals or from hospital teams, Social Services or the voluntary sector, particularly the Alzheimer's Society or Age Concern.

For younger people with dementia the memory clinic therefore represents an important avenue into getting help.

The Cerebral Function Unit (Robert Baldwin)

The Cerebral Function Unit (CFU), headed by Professor David Neary (see also Chapter 2), has for many years been the main local resource for the diagnosis of dementia in younger people living in Greater Manchester. This remains true but as Sean Page has pointed out another route is via the Memory Clinic. These services are not in opposition. Each offers different pathways to accessing services. What is vital for the development of local services for younger people is that there are clearly specified channels so that a diagnosis can be made with the minimum of delay.

The CFU (and units like it, for example, as described by Ferran et al, 1996, in nearby Liverpool) operates within a more traditional specialist medical-neurological framework. Its core membership comprises neurologists, neuropsychologists, a social worker and administrative support, often with a number of doctors and other professionals in training in attendance for whom it is an important training opportunity. Patients, who are referred by other specialists, such as psychiatrists but also primary care physicians, attend for a half day during which they receive a comprehensive diagnostic evaluation. This includes a history, mental state examination, physical evaluation and detailed neuropsychological testing (Chapter 2).

Neuroimaging is organized separately but wherever possible the referrer is given a provisional diagnosis within a few days. A follow-up visit is arranged after the neuroimaging is available at which a definitive diagnosis is given to the person affected.

Because dementia in a younger person can present differently and be caused by conditions rarely met by older adult services (Chapter 1), it is vital to have local expertise on hand. The exact solution will vary from locality to locality and not all regions of the UK have a service like the CFU. However, it is important to identify a neurologist who has an interest in dementia in the locality where the younger persons service is to be based.

The Old Age Psychiatry Service (Robert Baldwin)

Old age psychiatry (OAP) is a relatively new specialty in the UK. In many countries there is no special provision for older people with dementia, never mind younger ones. OAP services are charged with the assessments and management of mental health disorders among older people, usually defined by the rather arbitrary cut-off of 65 years. Services comprise a range of community, inpatient and day-patient services. Increasingly, the emphasis is on community care and the hub of many services is the Community Mental Health Team. This comprises (ideally) the relevant disciplines such as psychiatrist, nurses, psychologist, occupational therapist, speech and language therapist, physiotherapist, etc., often with sessional commitments from some of the shortage disciplines.

Over recent years two developments have taken place which have an impact on younger peoples services. The first is the growth in the number of psychiatrists choosing to train in the specialty and the increase in training standards. In an earlier survey conducted within Manchester before the advent of a younger persons service, Allen and Baldwin (1995) found that the local Old Age Psychiatry Service did not match the CFU with respect to its thoroughness of diagnostic evaluation of younger people referred for assessment, although it did offer more comprehensive aftercare. The authors' advice was to seek a neurological opinion from a physician with expertise in diagnosing younger people with dementia. Since then, the rise in training standards and the greater availability of neuroimaging means that this advice may no longer be valid—many old age psychiatrists are now trained to undertake detailed assessment of a younger person with dementia. However, these are issues that must be tackled locally.

The second development is the NSF for Older People, which as already mentioned, does incorporate services for younger people with dementia. Although not prescriptive, this will often be interpreted locally as meaning OAP services will take the lead. An issue that younger persons dementia services must address is what happens when the individual is no longer young, specifically, when he/she reaches the age of 65. There is no right or wrong answer, but in the Carisbrooke Manchester service the decision was taken, with the agreement of local OAP services, that transfer would take place at age 65. The main reason for this was pressure to take new referrals. The process now is that within three months minimum of the younger person reaching their 65th birthday, a care planning meeting will be held and arrangements made for a gradual handover of care. The principle is to allow sufficient time for the person to take in new faces and new premises. Following transfer the handover period usually lasts for up to three months.

References

Allen NH, Baldwin RC (1995) The referral, investigation and diagnosis of pre-senile dementia: two services compared. *Int J Geriatr Psychiatry* **10:** 185–190.

Crook T, Bartus RT, Ferris SH et al (1986) Age associated memory impairment: proposed diagnostic criteria and measures of clinical change. Report of a National Institute of Mental Health work group. *Dev Neuropsychol* **2:** 261–276.

DoH (Department of Health) (1998) *Saving Lives: Our healthier nation. A contract for health. A consultation paper.* London: DoH.

DoH (1999) *A National Service Framework for Mental Health: modern standards and service models.* London: DoH.

DoH (2001) *A National Service Framework for Older People: Modern standards and service models.* London: DoH.

Donaldson C, Burns A (1999) Burden of Alzheimer's disease: Helping the patient and caregiver. *J Geriatr Psychiatr Neurol* **12:** 21–28.

Ferran J, Wilson K, Doran M (1996) The early onset dementia: a study of clinical characteristics and service use. *Int J Geriatr Psychiatry* **11:** 863–869.

Gilleard J, Keady J (1998) Living with the early experience of Alzheimer's disease: the perspective of the person with dementia. In *Life After Diagnosis: A report on meeting the needs of people in the early stages of dementia.* Alzheimer Scotland Action on Dementia, Ch. 2.

Hassiotis A, Walker Z (2001) Setting up a memory clinic. In Walker Z, Butler R (eds) *The Memory Clinic Guide.* London: Martin Dunitz, Ch. 2.

Luscombe G, Brodaty H, Freeth S (1998) Younger people with dementia: diagnostic issues, effects on carers and use of services. *Int J Geriatr Psychiatry* **13:** 323–330.

NICE (National Institute for Clinical Excellence) (2001) *Technology Appraisal Guidance Number 19: Guidance on the use of donepezil, rivastigmine and galantamine for the treatment of Alzheimer's disease.* London: NICE.

Winning F (1998) Meeting the support needs of people with dementia. In *Life After Diagnosis: a report on meeting the needs of people in the early stages of dementia.* Alzheimer Scotland Action on Dementia, Ch 4.

WHO (World Health Organization) (1992) *ICD-10: The International Classification of Diseases and Health Related Problems.* Geneva: WHO, 10th rev. edn.

Wright N, Lindesay J (1995) A survey of memory clinics in the British Isles. *Int J Geriatr Psychiatry* **10:** 379–385.

chapter 13

Multiagency working

Michelle Murray

It has often been our experience that a diagnosis of dementia in working-age adults has enormous impact and far-reaching effects. The implications for the family, finances, employment and the future can seem insurmountable. When the person affected has a concurrent illness, such as human immunodeficiency virus (HIV), or alcoholism, the impact of a dementia can be complex, to the person, his/her carers, family and to service providers. Those affected require appropriate information, advice and support.

A knowledge and awareness of disease processes, the treatments available and emerging treatments are paramount. Working out the complexities of, for example, whether a person with acquired immunodeficiency disorder (AIDS) is losing weight because of systemic illness, comorbid depression or dementia-associated self-neglect will require practitioners from several agencies to work together.

HIV-associated dementia

There have been a handful of cases of persons with dementia associated with HIV/AIDS referred to the Manchester service at Carisbrooke. We have found them to present some of the most complex and challenging problems of any cases seen hitherto.

If cognitive symptoms arise it is essential to differentiate HIV brain impairment from opportunistic brain diseases (Kocsis, 1998). This is primarily because the latter are in the main treatable. It is important to also note that the person's condition will not necessarily deteriorate, especially in the early stages.

As has been outlined in Chapter 2, if dementia occurs, the main features conform to a subcortical pattern of illness: mental slowing, poor concentration and inefficient memory, along with apathy in some cases and disinhibited behaviour in others. The introduction of the combination therapies in 1996 has seen a decrease in mortality, permitting many individuals to carry on their lives with an undetectable viral load. Unfortunately, as with all medicines, these therapies cannot be tolerated by everyone. Compliance is a further issue. When a person with HIV has dementia, treatment compliance poses additional difficulties. Working collaboratively with other specialist services ensures that individuals and their families, carers or partners receive essential information, support and advice from the appropriate agencies at the right time.

Case study I

David, a 32-year-old, was referred to the Manchester service at Carisbrooke by a local nursing home which was having problems with his 'difficult behaviour'. David would scream very loudly and become verbally abusive towards staff. David was neglecting his personal hygiene and would spend most of the day lying on his bed, following which he would then spend much of the night awake.

At the initial visit, David was polite and cooperative. He gave a sketchy family history. Both parents were alive and well and had custody of David's 13-year-old son whose mother had died from AIDS three years earlier. David and his former partner had been drug misusers. Up until the involvement by the Carisbrooke Service, neither David's father nor his son had visited him since his admission to the nursing home. Staff from the local HIV liaison team felt that David was by now physically very unwell and that they would offer David and the nursing home continued support and advice regarding the treatment of his HIV. However, they were at a loss as to how to manage his behaviour.

The HIV liaison team had known David for six years and had extensive knowledge about him, including helpful information about his premorbid personality. The Carisbrooke specialist nurse facilitated a meeting with David, a nurse from the HIV liaison team and a member of the nursing staff of the nursing home. David felt that nursing staff often ignored him or tried to boss him. He felt that he had no privacy, and no one to talk to, saying that the majority of clients again were all too old to make friends with.

David also consented to a family meeting in order to encourage him to articulate his concerns to his family and to the nursing team. His mother, father and sister attended the meeting. Although David did not participate very much he appeared to listen to what family members and nursing staff from the home had to say. It became apparent that David's deteriorating illness was very distressing to his father and to his son and this was complicated further by their feelings at seeing him amongst much older people.

As a result of these meetings it was agreed that a family room would be prepared so that David and his family could meet away from the communal areas. Regular leave from the nursing home was also arranged so that David could visit his family at home, something that no one had made clear to the family could occur. The specialist nurse facilitated several more meetings with nursing home staff (both qualified and unqualified) in order to examine issues such as dignity, isolation and bereavement. She also met with David twice a month to give him an opportunity to talk. From this it was possible to feed back to the nursing home staff David's feeling that he had no control over his mortality and that he sometimes needed to vent his anger and frustration. Lastly, David continued to be visited twice-monthly by the HIV liaison team. As a result of these interventions, which had been coordinated by the specialist nurse from Carisbrooke, the problematic behaviour became less frequent.

Alcohol-related dementia

From discussions with other providers offering services to younger people with dementia around England it has become clear that there is controversy about whether there is such a thing as alcoholic dementia and even if there is whether it should be of concern to specialist dementia care.

Addressing the former issue, the brain pathology, cognitive changes and behavioural features associated with alcohol misuse have been outlined in Chapter 2. It seems reasonably clear that sustained heavy use of alcohol results in amnesic disorder and frontal lobe changes and that poor diet and self-neglect may exacerbate these effects.

As regards the second point of contention, working in an inner-city deprived area, it has been our experience that there is most definitely a high incidence of brain impairment due to alcohol misuse. As the Carisbrooke service is needs-led we took a decision as a team that each case referred to the service would be assessed individually on the basis of need and not merely diagnosis. However, if an individual continued to consume large amounts of alcohol or attended sessions at Carisbrooke in an intoxicated state we would discontinue the service, offer to point him/her in the direction of appropriate help and work with the local alcohol team to assist the person in reducing their alcohol intake. We find that some individuals can and do stop drinking, whilst others genuinely attempt to moderate their consumption. Hardest to help are those who live alone because their amnesia makes it difficult to change habitual patterns of behaviour.

Case study 2

Jeff is 56 years old. He was referred by the social work team from one of the local general hospitals. Jeff had been admitted to hospital following a collapse in the street. He was the youngest child of three and until this urgent hospital admission had been living with his elderly mother, following the break-up of his marriage six years earlier. He had not worked for the past three years because of his heavy drinking. He had not claimed any benefits or entitlements and instead had been living off his mother's limited income.

Jeff's mother wanted him to return home. However, other family members did not agree with this. They voiced concerns that Jeff became very verbally abusive towards his mother especially when she tried to stop him drinking. It was about this time that Jeff also developed alcohol-related seizures. Although he was prescribed medication, it became clear that he was unable to comply fully with it, not least because of his amnesia and lack of insight. He was also prone to falls and when his mother tried to help him she placed herself at risk of back injury. Throughout his time in the hospital Jeff refused to admit he had an alcohol problem. It was therefore agreed at a discharge planning meeting that Jeff should not return home to his mother.

Jeff was referred to Manchester's community alcohol service and a worker appointed to help him abstain from alcohol. Although Jeff had agreed not to return to his mother's home, there seemed to be few housing options for him. Living alone would certainly mean that Jeff would start drinking again and, of course, there was the added problem of his medication for seizures. Although he might have been placed in residential care this would result in him losing his independence.

Jeff was found accommodation with a family. This scheme, known as adult placement, offers patients or clients day care, respite or longer-term care in a family home. Jeff was also offered two days day care a week at the Carisbrooke younger persons service and was encouraged to visit his mother several times a week. He was given advice about benefits and finances. He became an active member of the allotment project (Chapter 5) and also baking and craft groups. Following discharge from hospital Jeff attended a clinic for his epilepsy, a weekly alcohol support group at Carisbrooke (Chapter 9) and was assisted with practical care by one of the Carisbrooke support workers on an outreach basis (Chapter 8).

This case again demonstrates how the younger persons service can offer strategic coordination of care in complex cases as well as offering some practical interventions.

Conclusion

In considering links with other agencies it is crucial to become actively involved in training. All members of the team have been required on occasions to provide training to other professionals in small groups and at larger-scale training events. These have varied greatly from students in all disciplines either in local colleges or on placement with the Carisbrooke service to large conferences. Clearly, one-to-one learning for carergivers and the younger person with dementia is another aspect of training.

Reference

Kocsis A (1998) *AIDS, Dementia and HIV Brain Impairment.* AVERT AIDS Education and Research Trust.

chapter 14

Views of users and carers

Emma Shlosberg, Caroline Browne and Alice Knight

As has been discussed earlier (Chapter 9) much of the research on dementia up until the late 1990s had focused on the impact and associated stress of caring for a relative with dementia. There has been limited research aimed at understanding the perceptions, views and experiences of those people with a diagnosis of dementia.

In England, the National Strategy document, *Caring for Carers* (DoH, 2000) stated that mental health services will be expected to plan improvements to services for carers, and highlighted the need to involve them in this process. To date, research assessing satisfaction with existing resources and service systems for younger people with dementia has largely confirmed carer and user dissatisfaction. Sperlinger and First (1994) described the stress caused to carers in trying to 'fit' younger people with dementia into day care services designed for older people. Similarly, Quinn (1996) found that carers found day care and respite services to be inappropriate because of the age of the person with dementia.

We simultaneously describe a research project of user satisfaction and one of carer satisfaction, along with an evaluation of the day care services provided by the Manchester Carisbrooke service. In keeping with a person-centred approach to dementia care (Chapter 9), the data is qualitative in nature, allowing the finer details of the subjective experiences of those people attending the day centre to be illuminated and prioritized.

Research projects

Research design

The aim was to elicit subjective experiences of users and carers and to explore in detail their views of the service. The resulting information was examined using interpretative phenomenological analysis (IPA). This approach is phenomenological in that it is concerned with an individual's personal perception or account of an object or event, but it is interpretative in that the researcher's own conceptions are required in order to make sense of the other's personal world (Smith et al, 1999)

Recruitment of participants

A potential group of service users was identified by the team (the criteria being that they could give information without becoming unduly upset), and of these, ten were chosen at random by a researcher. For the carers, the research was introduced at a carer support group. This meeting also acted as an informal focus group in which carers were given the opportunity to suggest any particular topics that they felt would be important areas for discussion. The researchers then considered these suggestions when designing the interview schedule. Approximately 30 carers currently make use of the service in some way and five carers participated. They were chosen because they had made, or were currently making, considerable use of the service.

Interview schedule

Open-ended questions were used to allow the participants to expand on each question as they wished. Prompts were developed in order for the interviewer to clarify any responses or expand on any questions if necessary. The initial interviews acted as a pilot in order to identify and prepare for any potential practical and process issues. Two separate interview schedules were designed:

1   *Users*. Questions focused on initial impressions of the service, views on access, information sharing, staffing issues, complaints procedures and activities.

2   *Carers.* The focus group allowed carers to be consulted in designing the interview schedule in an attempt to ensure that the
content of the questions would be meaningful to participants. The
manager of the service was also consulted during this process.
Questions focused on initial impressions of the service, views on
the day care facility and carer support group, and overall satisfaction. Questions were also asked about suggestions for future services.

Procedure

Users of the service were approached by a familiar member of the day
care staff team and asked if they would be willing to participate in the
survey. All the user interviews took place at the Carisbrooke centre,
whereas most of the carers chose to be interviewed at home. All the
participants were provided with an information sheet, which included
information about the interviewer, the rationale for the study, issues of
confidentiality and the interview procedure. Participants were
informed of their rights to withdraw at any time. They were also
asked to complete a consent form, stating that they wished to participate and that they were willing for the interview to be audio-recorded.
Recordings were later transcribed by the researchers.

Demographics

The ten users comprised six men and four women whose ages ranged
from 42 to 64 years. Four had a diagnosis of alcohol-related dementia,
four dementia of the Alzheimer's type and two vascular dementia.
They had been attending the centre from three months to four and a
half years. Four of the participants also received some outreach
support from the day centre. Participants attended day care from one
day to three days per week.

   Of the five carers one was male and the remainder female, with a
mean age of 57 years (range 52–60 years). All participants were the
spouse or partner of the person with dementia, and all were the
primary caregivers. Four carers lived with the person they cared for.
The husband of the fifth carer had recently moved to a nursing home.

All were white. Four of the people being cared for had Alzheimer's disease and one had vascular dementia. The time since diagnosis ranged from two to five and a half years, and the length of time participants had been using the service ranged from one to five years. Four of the people being cared for received day care at the Carisbrooke centre twice a week. One attended for one day a week. Four carers also had some experience of the outreach service provided by the service.

Analysis

The resultant transcripts were analysed individually using IPA, which incorporates a form of content analysis (Smith et al, 1999). The researcher carefully and repeatedly read each of the transcripts, noting down initial thoughts and attempting to understand what each participant was saying. Emerging themes and key issues were extracted and those relating to each other were grouped together. A consolidated list of superordinate and subordinate themes, reflecting shared aspects of experience for all the participants eventually emerged. In order to reduce the likelihood of researcher bias influencing the findings, a second researcher conducted a coding check, by sorting a list of random quotes made by participants into the identified themes. The themes were perceived to be robust and independent from one another and it was agreed that they accurately captured the participants' views.

Themes

The following themes are those which participants expressed most consistently. Of necessity, the findings are abridged but it is hoped that the selected quotes capture the experiences.

User satisfaction
Accessibility

All participants stated that they did not have any problems in getting to or into the centre once they arrived. It was, however, recognized that taxis were occasionally late.

Sometimes you get an odd taxi where they want a cash job rather than an account job. They're pretty regular the drivers, I know most of them now.

Involvement

Participants stated that they do have the chance to ask questions or get information when they are at the centre.

If there are any questions you can see one of the girls.
There have been a number of questions I've asked and I've got helpful answers.

All participants stated that they would complain about something if they wanted to.

If there are any questions you can see one of the girls.

Participants stated that they get involved in decisions that affect the service.

Sometimes we have discussions about things we could be doing and the majority gets the vote.
A suggestion was made for improving the situation.

If there is an open policy where you could feel comfortable in coming forward and saying 'I think I could improve this and what about this?', and coming up with ideas. There ought to be some sort of a sheet where you can write some ideas down, you know as a suggestion.

Relationships

The results were unanimous, stating that staff provide excellent help and support.

> *The staff are all great people.*
> *They've always got time for you.*
> *They go out of their way to try and get stuff for you. They're all very helpful.*

Despite the obvious appreciation of the staff, participants stated that there was not enough staff.

> *Sometimes there is never enough staff, especially if some people have to go out.*
> *If they want to improve the service an extra person or two might be useful.*

Participants stated that they enjoyed spending time with other users of the service.

> *It's nice to know you are not on your own.*
> *You get to meet quite a lot there that are probably in the same boat.*
> *It's one happy family.*

Accommodation

Half of the participants highlighted the inadequacies of the building.

> *We need a bigger one . . . I think we'd be able to do more to be honest with you.*
> *When there is a lot that come in it can be a bit crowded.*
> *It would be good if it was on the ground floor.*

Expectations and impressions

Expectations of the service varied.

> *I just felt at home straight away.*

I was frightened, very frightened.
I didn't come for six months. Once I came I couldn't keep away.
Can't keep away now unless I'm really ill.

Half of the participants stated that the centre was not like they thought it would be.

It was a pleasant shock to see people my own age and younger and I could relate to them.
It was good and perhaps not completely as I wanted or expected but certainly a damn sight better when I got in here than what I was led to believe it would be like.

Overall satisfaction

All participants could name things they enjoyed about the centre.

It's a home from home.
The relaxed air about it.
Meeting people in the same boat as you.
The fact that we see the same faces, that is reassuring

Suggested changes

More organized trips.
I like cooking. We don't seem to do a lot of that.

Impact on their lives

All participants stated that the centre had made their lives better.

I find that I've got more confidence in myself. I'd no confidence at all until I came here.
It gives me an interest back . . . Meeting new people.
Oh yes, it certainly gave me a brighter outlook and made it something to look forward to in the day.

Participants were asked if they were doing things that they would not do if they did not attend the centre.

I go out and I didn't go out before.

I am, yeah. Playing snooker, a game of cards or a game of dominoes. That's the time I'd be stuck at home doing nothing.

Additional information

Participants were given the opportunity to comment on anything that had not been discussed. One person made a request for respite care to be offered by the centre and another for more activities to be offered.

Carer satisfaction

Initial expectations and impressions

Carers reported feeling uncertain and apprehensive about whether the service would be helpful.

I thought when I first saw it [name of service user] would last one day ... that it wouldn't be her scene, that people were far more severely disabled than she was and that would upset her.

However, feelings of apprehension quickly faded as the service user settled in.

Now she is clearly one of the group ... She loves it, it's the highlight of her week.

Carers experienced a great sense of relief during the initial stages of using the service.

I was just happy that someone was helping me and, you know, giving us something.

Relationships

(a) Between service users

It was perceived that service users enjoyed spending time together and cared about one another.

[name of service user] took the trouble to write me a little note to say she was worried about [carer's husband] because he wasn't very well . . . now I mean that is so kind isn't it? . . . she took the trouble to send this note . . . I think that shows that they care about each other.

(b) Between staff and service users

Relationships were seen in a particularly positive light. Carers felt that staff respected service users and treated them with kindness and dignity.

The girls at Carisbrooke know . . . he's not a number, he's not just somebody who goes to the clinic once a fortnight or once every six months . . ., they know his silly little gags . . . and that's the nice thing about it, they're treating them still as individuals and not as well 'this man's got dementia so let's treat them all the same'.

(c) Between staff and carers

Carers felt extremely well supported by the staff team.

If you've got any problems, if you ring up and they can help, they do . . . and they are very understanding . . . and I think that goes a long way.

(d) Between carers

The opportunity to meet and share experiences with other carers at the carers support group was highly valued.

To meet other carers is a great support, to find that other people get just as tired or just as impatient.

However, one carer who chose not to attend the group commented:

I feel I can relax better with people who are maybe not in the same situation, probably I'm a bit too selfish to also want to listen to their woes.

187

Building self-confidence

Carers felt the service had been instrumental in helping the person with dementia to rebuild lost confidence.

> *He described it as the last two years he's been going through a dark tunnel where he's had everything taken away from him and lost control . . . and now he feels he is coming out again, he's getting his confidence back . . . and I have to think that's partly due to Carisbrooke as well.*

Meaningful activity

Carers felt the activities provided at day care were meaningful and enabled service users to maintain individual interests.

> *He used to bring things home he'd made or been helped to make with great pride and I think he enjoyed that.*

Accommodation

The accommodation in which the day service is housed was severely criticized.

> *For active young people you need the space.*

Transport

Dissatisfaction was expressed with using taxis to transport service users to and from Carisbrooke. It was perceived that a minibus, with a staff member present, would be safer and a great asset to the service.

> *I think if they had a minibus they could pick so many up . . . and one of the staff could drive it . . . I think it would be a fantastic thing and it would get them out a lot more.*

High quality staff

Carers repeatedly emphasized how satisfied they were with the quality of the staff working in the service. Staff were perceived to be knowledgeable, skilled, caring, humorous and positive in their attitude to dementia.

The way the girls work, it's like a networking system . . . I don't know how they do it, they're so coordinated somehow.

Time for the carers

The importance of allowing time for the carer also surfaced as a theme. Carers felt they could relax in the knowledge that, whilst at day care, their spouse or partner was in safe hands.

I know they are looking after him . . . I don't worry while he's there, never...you can be normal for a day, just be yourself and do what you want to do for one day.

Another carer felt the service had enabled him to keep working.

I need to work for several reasons, not least my own well-being.

Improving and developing services

Frustration over lack of resources emerged as a theme. Carers felt extremely aware of the lack of resources available to the service and unanimously expressed frustration about this.

They do need bigger premises . . . when they get all the patients in there, it's not fair to them and it's not fair to the patients.
It should be available for more people . . . many more people, much bigger premises.

The need for a flexible, seamless and integrated service, including a respite facility, was also raised. All participants expressed a wish for the service to extend in such a way that it could also offer age-appropriate respite care. Carers also felt that the service could be more flexible, in order to enable carers to continue working.

Conclusion

Several consistent themes emerged from the interviews. These are thought to reflect participants' shared experiences of the service. The overall perceived strengths of the current service are the relationships between staff, service users and carers, the meaningful nature of day care activities and the fact that the service caters specifically for the needs of younger people. Perceived weaknesses are the cramped and inappropriate accommodation, the use of private taxis to transport service users to day care, the lack of flexibility in the day care service and the need for increased service provision and more staff. The results of both surveys highlight the fact that the limited service available is a great success, but in need of development, notably in terms of extra personnel and a larger physical resource.

The qualitative approach used in this research allowed the participants to guide the discussion and allowed the researcher to flexibly explore in-depth issues which were of paramount importance to the carers. The usefulness of the approach is evident in the themes elicited. Whilst some of these were governed by the questions on the interview schedule, others were spontaneously generated by carers.

A major theme of relationships emerged from interviewing both users and carers and the topic of meaningful activity consistently arose too. Within these themes, it was recognized that service users were treated as individuals and it was recognized that each service user has different interests and a unique identity. These observations reflect the key principle of the recent culture of person-centred approaches to dementia care (Kitwood and Bredin, 1992) and differ from the traditional medical framework, which focused more on the diagnosis and extent of neuropathology.

The two surveys were based on the experiences of a small number of both carers and users of the Carisbrooke service. The representativeness of the findings could therefore be questioned. Despite the small sample size, the areas of desired change that emerged reflect issues that have been highlighted at a national level. The need for services to be organized in a flexible way so that carers can continue to work was emphasized in the recent National Strategy document *Caring for Carers* (DoH, 2000). The need for age-appropriate respite services has also been highlighted (Chapter 1). As the carers and service users were all white, there was no opportunity to address whether the service is responsive to the cultural diversity of its users.

Within the theme of initial impressions and expectations, users and carers were found to be initially apprehensive about using the service. It may be that people have incorrect perceptions about the service and lack knowledge about what to expect. If this is the case, providing the right kind of information may alleviate anxieties and result in more people benefiting from the service.

During the course of the interviews, users and carers suggested areas to improve the service. Several of these did not rely on a large increase in resources and we plan to incorporate them into the service over the coming months.

Results of both surveys have been circulated to managers and other staff involved in this process, as it is essential that the views of users and carers are considered and acted upon in any decision-making regarding future service development. It is also envisaged that work of this nature will be ongoing in that user and carer consultation will become a routine part of the service.

References

DoH (Department of Health) (2000) *Caring for Carers. The National Strategy.* London: HMSO.

Kitwood T, Bredin K (1992) *Person to Person*. Loughton: Gale Centre Publications.

Quinn C (1996) *The Care Must be There: Improving services for people with young onset dementia and their families*. London: The Dementia Relief Trust.

Smith JA, Jarman M, Osbourn M (1999) Doing interpretative phenomenologi-cal analysis. In Murray M, Chamberlain K (eds) *Qualitative Health Psy-chology. Theories and Methods.* London: Sage.

Sperlinger D, First M (1994) The service experiences of people with presenile dementia: a study of carers in one London borough. *Int J Geriatr Psych-iatry* **9**: 47–50.

chapter 15

Planning services for younger people with dementia

Michelle Murray and Robert Baldwin

Principles of service development

The Alzheimer's Society have outlined ten key messages in service development for younger people with dementia (Alzheimer's Society, 2001). These are:

1 *Seek the views of younger people with dementia.* Include younger people with dementia in the process of planning and evaluating services wherever possible.

2 *Use carers.* Carers have played a crucial role in raising awareness and campaigning. Their voice is very powerful in communicating the realities of existing support, lobbying politicians and service providers.

3 *Introduce organizational changes.* The introduction of named workers and referral pathways can make a significant impact on the quality of services for minimal cost. Specialist services can suffer from a lack of referrals if these structures are not in place.

4 *Involve people capable of effecting organizational change in the process.* Local politicians and leading doctors can play an important part in restructuring services.

5 *Be clear about where ongoing referrals will come from.* Ensure that the relevant people know what your service offers. Links with diagnostic services and commissioning agencies are vital.

6 *Look at the strengths in current provision and develop around them.* If there is no new money available adapt existing services— the service could be structured differently to reflect the needs of younger people (e.g. training could be offered).

7 *Learn from other people.* Make links with existing services and regional groups with a specific interest in younger people with dementia. (*see Appendix 2, Useful contacts*).

8 *Do not spend time surveying the needs of younger people with dementia.* Identifying where younger people are and developing a structure that directs people to appropriate professionals and services is a more useful exercise.

9 *Getting a service off the ground can be a long and frustrating process.* Keep people informed of developments to maintain their interest and support. Regular awareness-raising events and public meetings can also keep the momentum going.

10 *You will be under constant pressure to justify your service.* Keep the profile high—talk about your service, evaluate it, innovate.

Planning services

No matter how good the specialist service is for younger people, those who need it will not be referred unless the links with primary care have been thought through. The Alzheimer's Society (2001) recommends:

■ a focus on training primary care teams about dementia in younger people,
■ the need for clear referral pathways from primary care to specialist assessment,
■ the development of good practice guidelines.

Table 15.1 Preliminary data for planning a service

- Obtain local prevalence figure (see text)
- Estimate diagnostic heterogeneity (e.g. alcohol-related and vascular dementia)
- Identify lead consultant
- Identify lead nurse
- Identify local relevant resources (e.g. welfare and benefits advice)
- Identify and involve key stakeholders

To these may be added that the recent development in England of Primary Care Trusts (PCTs) affords an opportunity to strengthen liaison with primary care and to argue for funds, as in time, PCTs will control the majority of finances.

In planning a service (Table 15.1), it is important to know roughly what numbers of younger people to expect. In the past, we would have recommended a local survey but recent epidemiological surveys have rendered this unnecessary, at least in the UK. By accessing a website: (http://www.alzheimers.org.uk/ypwd/Statistics.htm), the number of those who have dementia in younger life can be determined for a given UK region or large town. As a caveat it is important to take into account local factors as the figures are most reliable for Alzheimer's dementia. For example, in Manchester we have a high demand from individuals with alcohol-related and vascular dementias.

It is neither necessary nor desirable to replicate generic services. For example, if there is a good welfare rights and benefits service then it should be accessed. Prior to establishing any new service it is important to identify the key stakeholders and involve them in a project development group. Stakeholders include members of the local PCTs, carers and social services personnel.

Once a development group has done its work the service will need a multiprofessional steering group that meets regularly—for example, in Manchester this meets every two months. In a multidisciplinary team it is important to delineate who is managerially responsible for the service and who will provide the professional support to individual staff. For example, an occupational therapist may be managerially responsible to the overall business manager of the department in which the service is based (e.g. old age psychiatry), but may receive professional supervision from someone in a neighbouring Trust.

We have found that regular strategy days, perhaps twice-yearly, in which all users and staff are involved are very useful. With good facilitation these can lead to important service developments.

Table 15.2 summarizes some of the practical issues that must be addressed before setting up a new service. A single point of access should be arranged (e.g. a telephone number). Agreement must be reached about the process of making a diagnosis, for example, by neurological services or memory clinic.

Identifying medical responsibility

Protocols should be developed regarding respite care and acute admission on psychiatric grounds. Because patients with dementia in younger adulthood are often quite fit physically, an old age psychiatric ward may not be the best place to admit a disturbed younger person with dementia. There must be clear agreement over admission rights and medical responsibility when patients are admitted in crisis.

Clear arrangements should be reached about medical responsibility for patients of the services. This is not necessarily straightforward as there are several options, at least in the UK. First, psychiatrists who treat working-age adults could take medical responsibility but this may be difficult as younger patients with dementia may not meet criteria for 'severe' mental illness, as required by the UK Care Programme Approach. Alternatively, an old age psychiatrist might assume responsibility, although the resources available may not be appropriate for younger people. A third option exists if there is a psychiatrist with dedicated time for younger people with dementia. Here, the

Table 15.2 Practical issues in planning a service for younger people with dementia

- Single point of access
- Clear arrangement and protocols about who makes the diagnosis
- Right of access to all existing relevant generic services
- Care coordination by a key worker
- Access to a reasonable range of specific services
- Clear protocols for respite care
- Clear protocols for emergency psychiatric admission

issue concerns the resources that the specialist psychiatrist has at his/her disposal. In the Manchester service, our experience can be summarized as follows. Patients with complex needs (equating to enhanced care under the Care Programme Approach) are best cared for by the psychiatric team dealing with working-age adults. Those whose psychiatric needs are not complex but whose medical condition is dominated by frailty, as in some cases of vascular dementia, are best catered for by old age psychiatric services. The final group comprising individuals without complex psychiatric needs and who are relatively medically fit, may benefit from a specialist service. However, the team must have sufficient resources to meet the needs of the individual. In the Manchester service at Carisbrooke, the typical profile of such a patient is that he/she has moderate cognitive impairment, no challenging behaviours, stable medical problems and is in need of day care and outreach services. Importantly though, in our view, a poorly resourced or embryonic service for younger people with dementia ought to consider very carefully whether it should undertake medical responsibility for younger patients. Ultimately, the issue comes down to negotiating local protocols that provide maximum benefit to the younger person.

Information

A good database of information is invaluable to a specialist service. We have listed the more important ones in Appendix 2. The Alzheimer's Society has web pages devoted to younger people with dementia and a range of useful material. CANDID (Counselling and Diagnosis in Dementia) (Appendix 2) has been established at the National Hospital for Neurology and Neurosurgery, London with the aim of increased accessibility to advice, diagnosis and counselling to the person with a young onset dementia, their carers and other health professionals. CANDID also offers information and education to increase the general awareness of the needs of the younger person with dementia for nurses, doctors, social workers and others working within this specialized area.

Conclusion

At the time of writing, the first full-time psychiatric consultant post for younger people with dementia has been advertised in the *British Medical Journal*. Although this may seem unattainable in many parts of the world, let alone the UK, it signals a recognition that specialist services are a reality. The aim of this book is to illustrate the ways in which such services may enhance care to a group of people who hitherto have received suboptimal care and to encourage service development locally, nationally and internationally.

Reference

Alzheimer's Society (2001) *Younger People with Dementia: a guide to service development and provision.* London: Alzheimer's Society (UK).

Geriatric Depression Scale, 15-item version

Instructions: Choose the best answer for how you have felt over the past week.

1. *Are you basically satisfied with your life?* **No**
2. *Have you dropped many of your activities and interests?* **Yes**
3. *Do you feel your life is empty?* **Yes**
4. *Do you often get bored?* **Yes**
5. *Are you in good spirits most of the time?* **No**
6. *Are you afraid something bad is going to happen to you?* **Yes**
7. *Do you feel happy most of the time?* **No**
8. *Do you often feel helpless?* **Yes**
9. *Do you prefer to stay at home, rather than going out and doing new things?* **Yes**
10. *Do you feel you have more problems with your memory than most?* **Yes**
11. *Do you think it is wonderful to be alive now?* **No**
12. *Do you feel pretty worthless the way you are?* **Yes**
13. *Do you feel full of energy?* **No**
14. *Do you feel that your situation is hopeless?* **Yes**
15. *Do you think most people are better off (in their lives) than you are?* **Yes**

Notes: (1) Answers refer to responses that score '1'; (2) ≥ 5 gives sensitivity of about 85% and specificity of about 75% for depression.

Appendix 2

Useful contacts

ALZHEIMER'S SOCIETY (UK)
The Information Officer
Younger People with Dementia
Alzheimer's Society
PO Box 6086,
Leicester
LE2 6WX, UK

Phone: 0116 288 2503
Email: ypwd@alzheimers.org.uk
Website: www.alzheimers.org.uk/ypwd/index.html

CANDID (Counselling and Diagnosis in Dementia)
The National Hospital for Neurology and Neurosurgery
8–11 Queen Square
London
WC1N 3BG, UK

Phone: 020 7829 8773
Website: www.candid.ion.ucl.ac.uk

FAMILY CAREGIVER ALLIANCE
690 Market Street
Suite 600
San Francisco
CA 94104, USA

Phone: +1 (415) 434 3388
Fax: +1 (415) 434 3508

E-mail: info@caregiver.org
Website: www.caregiver.org/
Factsheets on Alzheimer's disease and on-line support group for Huntington's disease:

CREUTZFELDT–JAKOB DISEASE SUPPORT NETWORK
Contact: Mrs Gillian Turner
National CJD Case Coordinator
Birchwood
Heath Top
Ashley Heath
Market Drayton
Salop
TF9 4QR, UK

Phone: 01630 673993
Email: cjdnet@alzheimers.org.uk
Website: www.cjdsupport.net

DOWN'S SYNDROME ASSOCIATION
155 Mitcham Road
London
SW17 9PG, UK

Phone: 020 8682 4001
Website: www.dsa-uk.com

HUNTINGTON'S DISEASE ASSOCIATION
108 Battersea High Street
London
SW11 3HP, UK

Phone: 020 7223 7000
Email: info@hda.org.uk
Website: www.hda.org.uk

Northern Ireland Huntington's Disease Association
Contact: Aoise Bradley
Department of Medical Genetics
Floor A, West Podium Extension
Tower Block, Belfast City Hospital
Lisburn Road
Belfast
BT9 7AB, UK

Phone: 028 9032 9241, ext 2255
Website: www.northernirelandhd.triopod.com

LAWNET LTD
93–95 Bedford Street
Leamington Spa
CV32 5BB, UK

Phone: 01926 886990

PARKINSON'S DISEASE SOCIETY (UK)
215 Vauxhall Bridge Road
London
SW1V 1EJ, UK

Phone: 020 7931 8080
Freephone helpline 9.30 am–6 pm weekdays: 0808 800 0303
Website: www.parkinsons.org.uk

PENUMBRA
Supporting the client with Korsakoff syndrome
Norton Park
57 Albion Road
Edinburgh
EH7 5QY, UK

Phone: 0131 475 2380

PICK'S DISEASE SUPPORT GROUP
Secretary
3 Fairfield Park
Lyme Regis
Dorset
DT7 3DS, UK

Phone: 01297 445488
Website: www.pdsg.org.uk

PSP ASSOCIATION (Progressive Supranuclear Palsy Association)
Gayton Manor
Gayton
Northamptonshire
NN7 3HE, UK

Phone: 01327 860299
Website: www.pspeur.org

Index

Note: References to tables are indicated by 't' when they fall on a page not covered by the text reference